MW00781993

NATURAL

Natural

Black Beauty and the Politics of Hair

Chelsea Mary Elise Johnson

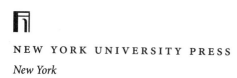

NEW YORK UNIVERSITY PRESS

New York

NEW YORK UNIVERSITY PRESS
New York
www.nyupress.org

Library of Congress Cataloging-in-Publication Data
Names: Johnson, Chelsea Mary Elise, author.
Title: Natural : Black beauty and the politics of hair / Chelsea Mary Elise Johnson.
Description: New York : New York University Press, [2024] |
Includes bibliographical references and index.
Identifiers: LCCN 2023058936 | ISBN 9781479814732 (hardcover) |
ISBN 9781479814756 (ebook) | ISBN 9781479814763 (ebook other)
Subjects: LCSH: Hairdressing of African Americans—Social aspects. | Hairdressing of
Black people—Social aspects. | African Americans—Race identity. | Black people—
Race identity.
Classification: LCC GT2295.U5 J65 2024 | DDC 391.5089/96073—dc23/eng/20240416
LC record available at https://lccn.loc.gov/2023058936

This book is printed on acid-free paper, and its binding materials are chosen for strength
and durability. We strive to use environmentally responsible suppliers and materials to
the greatest extent possible in publishing our books.

Manufactured in the United States of America

10 9 8 7 6 5 4 3 2 1

Also available as an ebook

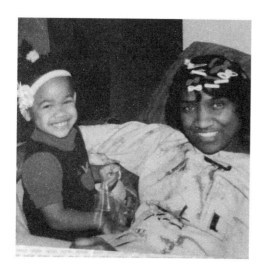

To my mom, my first and best example of Black feminism in action.

CONTENTS

FIGURES

PREFACE

My Hair Story

I received my first chemical relaxer when I was four years old in the form of a boxed kit of *Just for Me* relaxer that my mother bought for less than five dollars in the "ethnic aisle" at our local grocery store. We had vacation plans the following week, where I would be swimming every day, and my mom was determined to let me play in the water without spending hours detangling my thick, coiled hair each night. Neither of us considered that a restful holiday. And so, with hands covered in translucent, disposable plastic gloves always threatening to rip at the seams, she parted my hair in quarters. My forehead was thick with shine from the petroleum jelly that came with the kit, meant to prevent chemical burns. For the next fifteen years, I regularly relaxed my hair to keep up with my virgin "new growth," which would form a fluffy halo at my scalp, letting me know that it was time for my next treatment. During elementary school, my mom would braid my permed and hot-combed hair into neat cornrows, securing the ends with colorful plastic beads or bend-and-snap barrettes from the beauty supply store. Despite the heat and the chemicals, I thought of hair not as a burden but as a joy. It was a way for my mom and I to connect. I'd get her undivided attention for hours at a time on wash days. And on weekends, I'd spend an hour orbiting her, trying out new styles and testing my creativity. Sometimes, she'd even trust me with the scissors!

As the only Black girl in my class, I was on my own when classmates got curious about my hair. I remember field trips on the bus, where girlfriends would make sculptures out of my hair that stood stiff and straight, the overprocessing allowing each strand to defy gravity. I struggled to explain why it was not necessary for me to wash my hair every day, as they did, and why I'd add grease to my strands rather than obsessively shampoo it away. "It's not dirty, it's different," I'd explain, feeling unsure about whether this was true. Fortunately for me, my mom, like many Black parents raising children in predominantly white suburbs, was the queen of organizing everyday acts of resistance: she arranged to braid and bead two of my white kindergarten friends' hair as a form of cultural exchange. I remember feeling special when the braids slipped out of their silky hair overnight but mine stayed in for the next three weeks. (A decade later as a freshman in high school, I arranged my own "cultural exchange" and relaxed two of my white classmates' hair—this was the peak of the flat iron 'oos, and they were shocked that a permanent replacement for their flat irons existed. My mom was part horrified, part relieved that I somehow managed to avoid inflicting catastrophic chemical burns or baldness. The lesson? Not all forms of agency are resistant, productive, or wise.)

About once a year, when my mom could justify the expense, we would pay a family friend to style my hair into braided extensions. I loved those rare occasions, because I got to watch two or three Disney movies with the woman's daughters while she parted my scalp into a hundred tiny boxes, plaited each section until the synthetic hair reached my waist, and dipped the ends in boiling water so the plastic would melt just enough to keep the braid from unraveling. Little did I know, this delight in sisterly bonding through beauty culture was a tradition that went back generations, and made the Black beauty shop a central safe space for womanist organizing, a topic that we'll discuss at length in this book.

If ever I wore my relaxed hair "down" as a child, it was for picture day at school, weddings, Christmas card photos, or Easter service at the Southern Baptist church my family attended. Despite a lot of creative hair play during my childhood and adolescence, I was socialized to believe that long, straight hair was integral to preparing for important events, and that looking beautiful required hours of work and pain. In other words, I learned that hair straightening was central to *doing* Black girl-hood respectably. All the Black women in my life wore their hair straight, too—not only those in my mostly-white, middle-class neighborhood, but also those at my mostly-Black, working-class church, who came to service each week wearing their Sunday best, ready to be seen. By the time I entered middle school, I no longer remembered what my natural hair texture looked like. With few alternatives available in my personal life, on television, or in magazines, it never occurred to me to care.

It was not until I began undergrad at Spelman College, an Historically Black College for women in Atlanta, Georgia, that I began to think critically and strategically about my beauty routine. As upwardly mobile Black women in training, my classmates and I were taught through campus workshops that straight hair, navy blue suits, and Standard English were crucial to our future professional success. This was typical for many Historically Black Colleges and Universities (HBCUs) at the time: Hampton University famously banned students in its five-year MBA program from wearing locs or cornrows in 2001. Spelman lacked such an explicit policy, but almost all my classmates wore their hair straightened. Almost all of us had the "Spelman bob," a conservative, feathered hairstyle at the longest we could grow our hair before it broke off—usually near collar-bone length. I marveled at the many different techniques my classmates used to achieve silky hair when they walked across the Yard, the central area of campus that served as an unofficial fashion show. In Atlanta, widely hailed as the "Black hair capital" of the world, all techniques for styling curly hair textures were available at minimal cost. It was in Atlanta that I learned relaxed hair could have body and movement—what a marvel! Some of my classmates had ceramic flat irons that reached upward of 400 degrees Fahrenheit, while others wore wigs and weaves made from synthetic or human hair, installed at fifty-dollar weave shops in the West End or at the feet of enterprising classmates who put their skills to use to pay tuition, afford off-campus food, or buy a new club dress. I quickly learned by example, and soon became a master at wrapping my hair at night with satin scarves or looping my hair into perfect pin curls. My hair grew longer than ever with so much collective TLC.

While at Spelman, I met a pair of students at neighboring Clark Atlanta University who traveled back and forth to India importing bundles of unprocessed human hair to sell to discerning beauty connoisseurs in Atlanta. I took a trip to the duo's apartment and bought the rubber-banded ponytails of three anonymous persons, whose hair color matched each other's and mine well enough. I then sat at the feet of a weave master, who now works with celebrities like Naomi Campbell, Kim Kardashian, and Rihanna, to get the bundles installed. It was with this long, flowing weave that I won a campus homecoming pageant. My look was forever immortalized in a photo accompanying the school newspaper's front-page editorial, which criticized the idealization of women with light skin and long hair on HBCU campuses. I inadvertently became part of a long and extended debate about color hierarchies, texture privilege, and exclusionary beauty ideals in Black elite communities (see Craig, 2002). Confronting that unearned privilege made me burn with shame.

Alone in my dorm room one night, I stumbled upon the online blog *Black Girl with Long Hair*. The images I found of women with Bantu knots on their wedding day, before and after shots of teeny-weeny Afros (TWAs) turned massive halos, and aloe vera- and jojoba-coated curls were both inspiring and addictive. There were Black women of all skin tones and hair types choosing to embrace their natural hair textures. What was my hair texture? What did it feel like? And could I be as confident as these women on the internet? Privately, I decided to investigate what would happen if I skipped a relaxer that month. I rationalized that my hair was hidden anyway while cornrowed under my weave. What was the harm in a little experiment? This was 2010, and I eventually discovered that my personal natural hair journey was syncing up perfectly with what an emerging chorus of virtual hair gurus had termed the *natural hair movement*. I searched #naturalhair tags on social media and unearthed a host of other blogs, vlogs, and message boards filled with women who encouraged me to ditch my relaxer for good. After a couple of months, I was amazed to discover that I was growing ringlets of knitting-needle-size curls. I identified online influencers with my same hair texture, and these women taught me how to concoct mixtures of castor oil, honey, and flaxseed gel at home to avoid the parabens in store-bought products. Forum discussions suggested I swap the brands I grew up with for new haircare products for curls by Mixed Chicks on the West Coast or Miss Jessie's from New York. I learned a new set of terminology and came to understand that by growing out my relaxer, I was "transitioning."

The flourishing natural hair culture increasingly interested me. My changing body forced me to confront how uncritically I had internalized and embodied a belief that whiteness was more beautiful, more professional, more feminine. At the time, I was also coming to womanist consciousness while writing an undergraduate sociology thesis on Black women and the sexual politics of sport. My overlapping natural hair journey and journey as a sociologist inspired a critical interest in how race, class, and gender ideologies manifest themselves on and through the body. When I entered a doctoral program in Sociology at the University of Southern California, I chose to research how the natural hair movement might reveal what Black feminism looks like in a world that is increasingly global and commercialized. This took me on an unexpected journey from Los Angeles to New York, Cape Town to the Netherlands, and into virtual forums where women like me were coming to Black feminist consciousness as they discovered their bodies anew. In what follows, I describe the insights I garnered over the next six years, from 2013–2019. Through the voices, stories, and reflections of women who I met around the world, this book expands the ways that sociologists, feminists, and critical race scholars have understood the meanings of beauty politics, identity politics, and consumer politics. By fleshing out how the natural hair movement is changing what racial justice means today, I hope to provide readers with real life examples of how Black women's everyday practices have contributed to social change.

Writing this book was both enormously rewarding and frustrating. The natural hair movement is constantly evolving, with new businesses, films, websites, conflicts, hashtags, campaigns, and trends emerging all the time. I discovered so many interesting themes through this research process, and I struggled to find space to discuss them all. This was complicated by the fact that while this movement felt transformative for some, others felt excluded or devalued because of their class status, skin tone, global location, or hair texture. And as the world moved on from the 2010s to the 2020s, I noticed an opening up of the rigid natural hair politics of the previous decade—both on the internet and within myself. Trends and hearts are creating more space for aesthetic creativity and, dare I say, freedom in Black beauty spaces—spaces that are more inclusive and less critical of relaxers, flat irons, weaves, and wigs, and more understanding of the love for convenience, expression, and variety. I do my best to acknowledge, describe, and understand these contradictions and shifts in what follows. I would be so pleased if this book helps a new generation of Black women reflect on their beauty work with new interest, just as the bloggers, YouTubers, and natural hair organizers of the 2010s did for me.

Introduction

The New Natural Hair Movement

chop me from the neck up
& throw my head to the soft,
welcoming soil.

this is my ablution
permed edges,
burned forehead,
grown thick as wild crop after rain,
my hair isn't made of undulations,
so i blanketed my scalp in a white god,
pulled out each ancestor's song
until i met a new face in the mirror.
until this god harvested me with its greedy hands.
i was sewn a crown
of head sores & scorched earth & straw.
i looked kept & human now;
no one notices my split hoofs
or snout
or the deep bellow in my chest
when my fur is smoothed to someone's perfection.

this is my baptismal:

god of coconut oil
of Black castor oil

forgive me of my trespasses
bless my barren scalp

return me back to my beginning
forgive me for undoing your delicate labor
for opening myself to a false god
that will never love me

no matter how many times
I break myself in its image

each new curl howling a war cry
each howl an eviction notice

this is my ascension:

half rood, half glory,
all feral,
nothing that wouldn't snap
the teeth off a comb
& neck for good measure—
all I know is how to break soft things
i do not know any other way
than to be present
for this homecoming
i lift my hands in ceremony
to open my scalp for water.
for my curls to bloom onto themselves,
here: i am growing a forest on my head
here: i am renamed in an ancestor's hymnal.
listening to the rain for my Blkness,
i am a crown of what the heavens come to answer;

watch me king.
—I. S. Jones, "Wild Crown" (2016), permission granted by author

Everyone, everywhere, has a hair story.

I. S. Jones recited a poem about her hair story, "Wild Crown," to an enraptured audience at a 2016 Pride Week event I attended at a small performance café in downtown Brooklyn, New York. Given that only a handful of people in the audience appeared to be of African descent, "Wild Crown" might seem an unlikely choice for the occasion. And yet, those lucky enough to score a chair leaned in from their leather-cushioned perches. I sat cross-legged among the dozens of attendees in overflow spots on the floor, just inches before the small, raised stage. Though "Wild Crown" is not explicitly about gender identity or sexuality, Jones's narrative of coming out as her most authentic self despite cultural barriers to acceptance was familiar to many in the audience. Jones's performance was particularly conspicuous at this Pride event, which lacked any other explicit discussion of race as an identity that overlaps and intersects with gender and sexuality.[1]

I begin this chapter with "Wild Crown" because it so perfectly introduces the themes I'll unpack in this book. In the poem, Jones recounts turning away from the physical and emotional violence begot by chemical relaxers, and instead, deciding to "chop [herself] from the neck up," a reference to the "big chop," a rite of passage in the transition from relaxed to natural. She describes the process of discovering what her body naturally responds to and enjoys. She rebukes Eurocentric standards of beauty—"a false white god"—and speaks of embracing her ancestry from the inside out. Jones critiques hair straightening as a form of respectability politics—"i look kept & human now"—and mocks racist and sexist discourses that oppress Black women by likening them to beasts. Through poetic allusions to soil, forests, and flowers, "Wild Crown" reclaims the connection between Blackness and nature, reframing this association as a sign and source of Black resilience. Ultimately, Jones's natural hair journey becomes politically significant to her. Transitioning to natural hair feels empowering. And beyond the words of the poem, Jones's performance itself acted as a discursive tool to make space for herself in a political gathering that did not explicitly acknowledge her uniquely subjective, embodied experience as a Black woman whose intersectional identity seemed, until then, relegated to the periphery. In many other social activist contexts—like the Green Movement and the Movement for Black Lives—participants use natural hair to make space for, and call out how, the social world acts differently for and on Black women's bodies: bodies that are living, working, and loving at the bottom of intersecting race, class, gender, and sometimes sexual hierarchies. "Wild Crown" feels like a poetic distillation of this book.

Hair is not simply a biological fact. Hair can be cut, colored, dyed, covered, gelled, waxed, plucked, lasered, loc'ed, braided, relaxed, and many combinations of the above. Because of this versatility, visibility, and uniquely personal quality, it is the body's ripest material for creative self-expression.[2] As the most malleable part of the human body, hair almost always expresses social dynamics. Hairstyling practices demonstrate that large-scale social forces—political, economic, and ideological frameworks—are not divorced from the aesthetic and embodied choices that individuals make. Trends in the ways people manipulate their hair are always influenced by the social systems in which they live. Hair is also social in that, interpersonally, we "read" other people's hair for clues about where they stand in society and their political stance toward the world. Hair can signify age through graying or balding, health through hair loss or overgrowth, race through texture and color, and gender through the presence or absence of secondary sex characteristics and hairstyling. In many cultures around the world, hair is imbued with moral and spiritual significance; the symbolic value of hair is perhaps most visible in religious practices. Growing hair long is considered a sign of spiritual strength and commitment for Rastafarians and Sikhs, while hair-shaving rituals are incorporated during Hindu supplications to God. Covering hair signifies piety, obedience, and modesty for Muslim and Orthodox Jewish women. Hair was the ultimate source of strength for the Biblical figure Samson. Hair is, as sociologist Kobena Mercer puts it, "on the cusp between self and society, nature and culture."[3]

What does hair mean for Black women today? This book is about the hundreds of thousands, perhaps millions, of women of African descent who have transitioned out of chemically relaxed or thermally straightened hairstyles and embraced their naturally curly and kinky hair textures since the turn of the twenty-first century. Since hair is simultaneously gendered, racialized, and malleable, Black women's efforts to gain power, influence, adequate representation, and social mobility, can often be observed through the ways in which they style their hair. In the twenty-first century, these efforts have coalesced in the natural hair movement. In this book, I discuss how this movement has reimagined beauty, informed Black women's self-care practices, created novel spaces for cultural production, and catalyzed new forms of entrepreneurship within the Black beauty industry. *Natural* is about Black women's contributions to racial justice, gender equality, and the global economy through natural hair and Black beauty culture. Specifically, this book considers "going natural" as political resistance against a form of racism wherein white women's bodies are considered more beautiful, more professional, and more worthy of protection than other women's bodies.[4] Through the voices of some of these women, this research aims to contribute to how we understand the body as a vehicle for social change and as an influential factor in racial formation—a theory that sociologists Michael Omi and Howard Winant use to explain how racial categories, meanings, and power are created and transformed over time.[5] While people often think of race as a static concept, the natural hair movement shows how gender, colonial histories, and people's styling choices all influence what race means, what it looks like, and how it is embodied across time and space, echoing sociologist Shirley Anne Tate's apt observations that "Black beauty's Black Atlantic diasporic roots and routes has affected whole cultures as it has involved the shifting of socio-political not just aesthetic boundaries, transformed discourses and changed both individual and communal identities."[6] This is one story of how these changes are realized.

Black Bodies Matter

This book follows a full decade of organizing in the name of Black lives mattering, which has made abundantly clear how racialized state policies, economic arrangements, and cultural norms influence how Black people move through the world: how their bodies labor, how they are treated, the physical environments in which they live, and the degree to which they can express their individual agency.[7] That's why sociologists of embodiment theorize the human body as a "medium of culture," or a physical form through which social hierarchies, control, and etiquette are inscribed.[8] How Black bodies are seen by, are worked upon, and are treated by others can all be a starting place for discussing broader social dynamics in a specific place and time. After all, we move through the world *within* our bodies.

The loudest conversation about Black bodies has focused on state violence against Black men's bodies. However, social systems act on and alter bodies in a variety of ways—not only in the context of racism, but also in the context of patriarchy and capitalism. The term "gendered racism" captures the reality that women's bodies are assigned different levels of protection, value, and desirability depending on their perceived proximity to whiteness and wealth, thereby naturalizing and legitimizing inequality between women of different backgrounds.[9] Race always intersects with gender and class. Thus, women's bodies are interpreted, valued, and treated differently depending on their positions within a capitalist patriarchy. For example, through the late nineteenth century, white middle-class American women's status as dependents of their husbands or fathers prevented them from making decisions about their own monetary earnings, children's futures, and possessions, but Black enslaved women were *literally* property. Dating back to the transatlantic slave trade, the state and the media have deployed what Patricia Hill Collins calls "controlling images" of Black women—stereotypical and pejorative representations of Black women as oversexed jezebels, subservient mammies, and angry sapphires that justify their marginalization under capitalist, patriarchal white supremacy.[10] Beliefs about women's sexually seductive power are intensified for Black women and have been deployed by governments to rationalize forced sterilizations and punitive welfare policies, as well as to deny Black women's experiences of pain during childbirth.[11] Elite groups have represented Black women as the exemplary "Other" to white humanity to justify the use of Black women's bodies as unpaid chattel laborers and breeders for more slaves, and to shelter white men from legal penalties for raping Black women.[12] Racist tropes that Black women are inferior and subhuman have been mapped onto discourses about coily hair, which is routinely described as wild, exotic, or needing to be tamed.[13] These stigmas have persisted through to the present day. Moreover, stratified labor markets that usher many women of color into low-wage service work influence how Black women's bodies are used, what Black families consume, and how Black people style their bodies. The conditions of and stereotypes about Black women's bodies undermine them in ways unique from Black men and non-Black women. To analyze Black women's experiences—especially concerning their bodies and embodiment—from the lens of race, class, or gender alone would provide only a partial view of their unique experience at the intersection of multiple systems of social stratification. Black women's embodied experiences of enslavement, violence, citizenship, medicine, labor, love, and beauty cannot be understood without an intersectional lens.

Systemic gendered racism has both ideological and material consequences, and a Eurocentric beauty standard that idealizes long, straight hair is one manifestation of it. Black women face pressures to manage their embodied presentations-of-self due to their distance from valued forms of femininity and racist, sexist, and capitalist pressures that deem their bodies uncontrollable and uncivilized. Much intersectional research finds that economic constraints and racial domination make it harder for Black women to access the privileges afforded to those considered beautiful.[14] Light skin, European facial features, and slim body frames are resources—or feminine currencies—that are valuable in the

employment and dating markets.[15] Political scientists Jennifer Hochschild and Vesla Weaver find that "dark-skinned Blacks have lower socio-
economic status, more punitive relationships with the criminal justice
system, diminished prestige, and less likelihood of holding elective office
compared with their lighter counterparts."[16] Colorism, in addition to
what I'll call texturism, or the idealization of straighter hair,[17] intersect
with gender, as both light skin and long hair are considered not only
more beautiful, but also more feminine. Research also finds that skin
tone and hair texture stratify Black women's dating experiences and their
representations in the media.[18] Exclusionary beauty ideals are constantly
being reproduced by the fashion and entertainment industries. Representations of women's bodies as young, tall, thin, blonde, and light-
skinned within the mainstream media and advertisements continue to
perpetuate a white-centered ideal for feminine beauty, respectability,
and professionalism, constraining and informing women's options for
self-presentation.[19] For example, sociologist Ashley Mears describes
how representations in the entertainment and fashion industries, especially of women, are explicitly racially policed by advertisers, executives,
designers, photographers, editors, and modeling agents. These cultural
gatekeepers tend to exclude women of color from conceptualizations of
"high-end" in campaigns, fashion shows, advertisements, and ultimately
commonsense understandings of "taste." As a result, the commercial
fashion and editorial images that saturate everyday life participate in
a white-supremacist, capitalist patriarchal system that naturalizes and
reinforces social inequalities.[20]

Hair texture and style, in particular, are often used to measure Black
women's worthiness of economic, social, and cultural capital. As anthropologist and Black hair scholar Lanita Jacobs points out, "Black wom-
en's hairstyle choices are seldom just about aesthetics or personal choice
but are instead ever complicated by such issues as mate desire, mainstream standards of beauty, workplace standards of presentation, and
ethnic/cultural pride."[21] In other words, beauty standards have largely
served the interests of white people, men, and a capitalist market ever

threatening to leave non-compliant bodies behind. Hair straightening, adornment, cutting, covering, and styling are all strategies that Africana women have used to reimagine Black femininity and critique inequality through their bodies. Women's choices run up against social expectations, where she might be disciplined, celebrated, admired, surveilled, or rejected depending on the distance between her presentation-of-self and the presumed social norms. For example, when a Black woman chooses not to straighten her hair, her natural hair is often viewed by employers, educators, and romantic partners as an indicator of her inherent inclination to poverty, servitude, laziness, wildness, criminality, or backwardness, because straight hair has been tied to respectability and professionalism.[22] Black women's natural beauty has been denied by society, placing them beyond cultural conceptions of womanhood as represented by the media.[23] The result? Many Black women have been shamed into disciplining their bodies, using chemical relaxers and weaves to keep their jobs and appropriately perform heterosexual womanhood.[24] The treatment of Black women's natural hair as problematic demonstrates that "the allocation of power and resources not only in the domestic, economic, and political domains but also in the broad arena of interpersonal relations" is dependent upon "doing gender" per white standards.[25]

Gendered racism is so culturally entrenched that the notion that kinky hair textures should be straightened is often internalized by Black women themselves and transmitted across generations. Many Black communities consider hair relaxers (a chemical process that permanently straightens hair) both a rite of passage into Black womanhood and a sign of economic stability.[26] Because chemical relaxing in childhood was so widespread and ritualistic until the 2010s, most millennial and Gen X Black women were made unfamiliar with their own natural hair textures by adulthood. Ethnic studies scholar Ingrid Banks's interviews with Black American women in the 1990s reveal how understandings that wavy or curly hair is "good hair" and tightly-coiled hair is "bad hair" are learned by young children in schools, churches, and the home.[27] Some Black women and girls' feelings about themselves are formed in relation to these cultural discourses. Communications scholar Cheryl Thompson finds that Black and biracial Americans continue to engage in practices to align their appearance with white beauty norms and laments, "It is the 21st century, yet Black women are still struggling to meet this standard."[28] The "'Good Hair' Study," a 2017 study by the Perception Institute, investigated the prevalence and strength of this standard, measuring whether Americans hold any implicit or explicit bias toward Black women's natural hair, to understand the impact of hairstyle on how Black women are perceived by others and how they perceive themselves.[29] The Institute found that, while women of all racial backgrounds feel some level of anxiety about their hair, Black women experience higher levels of anxiety than others, and that Black women's anxieties around their hair are substantiated by white women's devaluations of natural hairstyles. Furthermore, a set of four studies and experiments by business management researchers Christy Koval and Ashleigh Rosette found that Black women with natural hairstyles were perceived to be less professional, less competent, and were less likely to advance in the job interview process than white women and Black women who wear their hair straight.[30] Regardless of race, most research participants showed implicit bias against Black women who wear their hair in textured styles. Banks further argues that kinky hair is so devalued in society and so significant to race, class, and gender identity that Black women are socialized into a collective consciousness around hair.[31] It is no wonder that "exploring how externally defined standards of beauty affect Black women's self-images, our relationships to one another, and our relationships with Black men has been one recurring theme in Black feminist thought."[32] Angela Davis, Phoebe Robinson, Toni Morrison, Chimamanda Ngozi Adichie, Zadie Smith, Alice Walker, and many other women writers across the African diaspora have made hair a recurring subject in their work.[33]

As so many iconic Black cultural artifacts show, individuals also have agency in how they navigate social structures. Elite groups do not have a unified gaze that maintains the total oppression of others; communities can and do redefine beauty, gender, race, and culture through hairstyling, creating spaces for the appreciation of difference. Race, as I see it, is also created, invoked, obscured, and reimagined through the self-representative choices people make. People can and do express, emphasize, or minimize signifiers of gender, race, and cultural identity through hairstyle, fashion, makeup, plastic surgery, and demeanor, and often in politicized ways. Embodiment is both the product of capitalist, white supremacist, and sexist systems *and* people's responses to and experiences of these systems. In other words, bodies are simultaneously objects and agents of racial formation. For Black women, body work is mutually informed by the pressures to avoid racist stigma and violence and the pleasures of securing social, cultural, and aesthetic capital.

As Black women enter community with one another, they often discover opportunities to create new meanings, narratives, and experiences of Black embodiment. For over a century, Black beauty shops have served as havens for conversation, sisterhood, and political organizing among Black women. Black feminist scholars have written extensively about how Black salons, hair shows and industry expos, and local meetups offer rare spaces for Black women to bond with one another, circumvent a racist job market to become economically independent, express creativity, politically strategize, and escape the stresses of work and family.[34] Furthermore, as scholars Kristin Denise Rowe and Omise'eke Tinsley point out, beauty culture holds special significance in Black queer communities, offering space for Black femininity and femme-ininity to share sisterhood and monetize cultural skills to create wealth and new cultural aesthetics.[35] I think back to my evenings in college spent at the feet of hairstylist Tokyo Stylez as she cultivated a beauty in, on, and through me with a skill so undeniable that her fame was inevitable. Comedian Phoebe Robinson aptly explains the subjective and collective aspects of Black hairstyling: "There is an element of play, like being a pop star who constantly reinvents her look. There's also a bond, a band of sisters, if you will, because when we see each other, we know *exactly* what it took to get our hair a certain kind of way."[36] Research on beauty pageants likewise documents how racially marginalized communities combat the systematic exclusion of non-white women from Western conceptions of beauty by organizing their own spaces, governed by their own beauty ideals.[37] While participation in beauty pageants might reinforce women's status as symbolic objects, Black-led pageants have also progressively rearticulated dominant Eurocentric standards of beauty to affirm darker skin, curlier hair, and fuller figures.[38]

The Natural Hair Movement

Despite the important havens of pleasure, experimentation, and joy that do exist, the natural hair movement took root and blossomed from relatively unlikely soil—a context characterized by gendered racism in relationships, in the job market, and in the media. Against an outpouring of white supremacist discourse and xenophobia across the United States and Western Europe in the 2010s and 2020s, natural hair has come to occupy an important place in Black women's identity politics across the *Black Atlantic*—what British sociologist Paul Gilroy terms the diasporic African community that spans North and South America, the Caribbean, West and Southern Africa, and Europe. Since kinky hair is a racialized feature, when women of color collectively celebrate the socially risky and unpopular choice to not straighten their hair, the body becomes a site of gendered racial resistance and contested meanings. Many of my interviewees have received criticism for their choice to wear natural hair, and they see this choice as the centerpiece of a political project—a way of "acting out" identity politics in contestation of a racialized desirability that devalues Black femininity. The natural hair movement illuminates both the pleasures of Black women's cultures and the specific violence of what communications studies scholar Moya Bailey calls "misogynoir," a particular form of anti-Black sexism directed toward women of African descent.[39]

An international community of women has made embracing their natural hair textures both a trend and an act of political agency over and against disparaging comments from family members, legally sanctioned dismissals from jobs, pat downs from airport officials, and pets from strangers that treat Black women like animals or public property. Across the new local, transnational, and virtual communities and industries they have built around natural hair care, these women have conceived of, named, and embodied the *natural hair movement*.[40] This book centers the women who participate in this movement, the spaces for sisterhood they have created, and their ventures for serving Black women's unmet demands for representation, political influence, and consumer options.

Natural hair communities are sizeable. CurlFest in Brooklyn, New York, and Taliah Waajid's World Natural Hair Show in Atlanta, Georgia both claim to host upward of 30,000 attendees at their annual events. These natural hair communities extend online, blurring the boundaries between physical natural hair meetups and digital natural hair forums. A quick YouTube search of "natural hair" yields millions of hits, and a Google search for blogs yields tens of millions more. At the time of this writing, #NaturalHair has been tagged in over fifteen million photos on Instagram. There are countless YouTube channels, Instagram accounts, Facebook groups, websites, blogs, Pinterest lists, and Tumblr archives dedicated to natural hair culture.

On- and offline natural hair spaces are neither static nor discrete. The natural hair movement follows not only the national, transnational, and digital migration of social media influencers, organizers, and lay participants, but also the circulation and exchange of products, hair care practices, politics, and Black feminist praxis among the ever-expanding community. With the rise of visually-oriented online social media platforms such as Instagram, long-standing circuits of cultural exchange among Africana women have expanded in the digital age. Through beauty "how-to" tutorials and grassroots content creation, natural hair has become the center of resistant and Black-affirming aesthetics and culture

FIGURE I.1.
Hundreds of
attendees gather
at a natural hair
festival. Author's
photo.

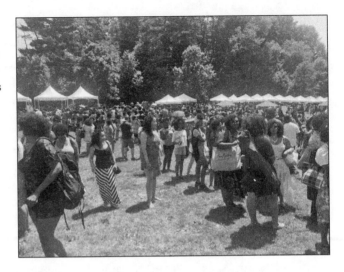

across the African diaspora. Geographically distant communities of Africana women collaboratively advocate for transitioning to natural hair through coordinated events like International Natural Hair Meetup Day, where communities from Japan to the Netherlands organize gatherings for local Black women to meet and discuss a coordinated program of topics. Alternative beauty pageants, like the one organized by performance artist Susana Delahante in Havana in 2015, which crowned seventy-two-year-old Felicia Solano's fluffy white Afro the winner, subvert exclusionary norms that measure women by their proximity to youth, whiteness, and wealth—and do so in front of a global audience of Instagrammers, Facebookers, and YouTubers armed with new images at their fingertips.

Such initiatives are so influential that wearing unstraightened, kinky hair is no longer a niche style among Black women. A new economy and culture around natural hair has caught the attention of mainstream media and transnational corporations, transforming relatively unknown vloggers into niche celebrities with sponsorships. Even pop culture's most iconic symbols for feminine beauty have responded to the natural hair movement's influence. In 2015, after decades of demands for more a realistic Barbie, Mattel introduced new dolls with darker skin tones and coily hair. That same year, Angolan model Maria Borges made head-lines for being the first Black woman to walk a Victoria's Secret runway show with her natural hair—a significant departure from the flowing extensions she wore in the previous two shows and the brand's signature long, wavy-haired representation of feminine desirability. In 2017, Miss Jamaica, Davina Bennett, became the first contestant with natural hair to reach the finals of the Miss Universe pageant and became a world-wide trending topic on Twitter because of her hair. The 2018 blockbuster film *Black Panther* was a celebration of natural hairstyles. Women in the fictional African nation of Wakanda sported shaved heads, Bantu knots, locs, braids, and Afros. One reviewer concluded that the film "weds a Black Nationalist aesthetic with an ethos of global kinship."[41] In 2020, the short film *Hair Love*, about a father learning to style his daughter's natural hair using digital video tutorials, snagged the Oscar for Best Animated Short. Around that same time, a new wave of public figures like singers Chloe and Halle Bailey, director Issa Rae, congress-woman Ayanna Pressley, actor Lupita Nyong'o, and later, former First Lady Michelle Obama helped expand the menu of styling possibilities for Black women represented in popular culture and politics to include loc'ed, shorn, braided, and twisted natural hairstyles. Then, major re-tailer Target created an entirely new front-facing display in the cosmet-ics section of its stores dedicated to showcasing products for naturally curly and kinky hair, many manufactured in small batches by emerging Black women entrepreneurs. Until recently, items for "ethnic" women had been marginalized to a small section at the end of the hair aisle or were omitted entirely from most stores depending on corporate analy-ses of neighborhood demographics. By creating a new area for healthy products to care for curls, major retailers were finally acknowledging that Black women are worthy of provision and that Black-owned com-panies are worthwhile investments.

I know some readers are probably cringing at my mention of Target. In a world where large corporations often co-opt social movements or make shallow, performative gestures to marginalized groups, it makes sense to be critical about any organizing where marketing, buying, and selling are central to the ways participants interact. Yet, as I will show, the natural hair movement *is* politically impactful even as it is undeniably a product of the neoliberal consumer context from which it emerges. It is both true that individual women turn to media representations and the market to remake themselves and to (re)claim Black women's natural hair as beautiful, *and* that natural hair culture tends to rely on the class privileges of internet access and disposable income to sample new products.

Unlike most beauty conventions that are primarily attended by industry professionals, natural hair shows are geared toward the lay consumer. Natural hair meetups are often held at parks or in exhibition halls at hotels, museums, or conference centers where stylists, beauty bloggers, and everyday women discuss hair politics, natural hair maintenance techniques, and the latest products hitting the market. Fashion shows, fitness classes, forums, and demonstrations operate concurrently in the same room, as women leisurely explore businesses' booths and listen to pitches from their representatives. Event attendees line up hours in advance, sometimes by the thousands, to receive SWAG ("stuff-we-all-get") bags filled with full-sized samples of creams and shampoos for naturally kinky hair that have been donated by event sponsors. The popularity and success of these events affirm that natural hair is both a movement and an industry. Despite this, Black women remain underserved by both the beauty- and green- consumer industries. Might there be space within neoliberalism for an anti-racist and feminist politics that not only allows for the pleasures of consumption and beauty, but also goes beyond individual empowerment to uplift Black communities more broadly? What draws millions of Black women to dedicate their bodies, time, and money to natural hair culture as opposed to another activity or political strategy in this historical moment? At present, the meanings and implications of Black women's organizing around natural hair remain under-interrogated.

The women you'll meet in this book resist the idea that natural hair is just a consumerist fashion trend, describing it as a political symbol, political act, and political experience. However, unlike during the 1960s and 1970s, wearing natural hair in the twenty-first century is not necessarily a signifier of Black Nationalist commitments. While some aim to change specific policies or institutional structures, most of the natural hair advocates I met work to transform white supremacist cultural notions that kinky hair is ugly, unprofessional, or unmanageable within Black women's own psyches. Alongside encouraging women of African descent to embrace the beauty in their kinks and curls, natural hair movement spaces provide practical information about healthy haircare practices and consumer options, and how to navigate pressures to straighten one's hair at school, at work, and in romantic relationships. Disseminating practical information is crucial, since many Black women have not seen their hair unstraightened since childhood and have long-relied on professional stylists for regular thermal presses and chemical relaxers. This dual goal of self-acceptance and knowledge distribution is exemplified by the massively successful, worldwide hair forum tour hosted by beauty blogger Taren Guy, entitled "Luv & Learn Your Beauty."

As a cultural phenomenon so global in scope that it engages participants across the African diaspora and forces established mainstream companies to reconsider their marketing tactics, the twenty-first-century natural hair movement begs deeper analysis. The simultaneous developments of the natural hair movement, social media technology, concern about the environment and climate change, and largescale anti-racist organizing and mobilization prompt urgent questions that allow us to move critical race and feminist theories in new directions: How are women of African descent reproducing, negotiating, and challenging ideas about beauty, race, and gender through natural hair? How do location and historical context shape what natural hair means to individual women and their communities? How does the current commercialized neoliberal context constrain, enable, and inform Black women's beauty practices and their meanings? And how does a curl become a movement?

I explore these questions through conversations with women in the United States, South Africa, Brazil, and the Netherlands, following them into their homes, their salons, their meetups, and their digital forums. I describe what these women say it feels like to challenge stereotypes about Black hair that they've internalized, that their communities uphold, and that the mainstream media perpetuates through exclusionary, white-centered representations of beauty and professionalism. I describe how Africana women are using natural hair to write new narratives—new articulations of their personal and collective visions for racial freedom, upward mobility, and women's empowerment. I engage debates about the potential for consumer politics to have positive social and individual effects by empirically investigating how women of African descent living in the twenty-first century experience consumer-based natural hair politics in their everyday lives. I examine the motivations of several natural hair entrepreneurs who use embodied knowledge gained from playing with—and caring for—kinky hair to create lucrative and rewarding haircare ventures they view as politically transformative. I show that the natural hair movement's focus on emotion, interpersonal relationships, and consumer options challenges sociological understandings about the defining features of a social movement, and that these theories expand when we take Black women's perspectives and lived experiences seriously. I also describe how transnational flows of people, products, practices, and politics shape the natural hair movement and advance intersectional critiques of the state, androcentric activist discourses, and the political economy. Focusing on where and how conversations about natural hair are taking place, as well as who is allowed and encouraged to participate in these conversations, I address the influence of Black women's changing beauty practices on their relationships with their bodies, in the virtual, global, and entrepreneurial marketplace, and among each other. The interviews, media analyses, and observations presented in *Natural* highlight the gendered dimensions of racial formation and reveal that racial projects draw from women's interrelated experiences of private, collective, and transnational violence and pleasure across the Black Atlantic. Africana women are imagining, expressing, and creating social change through their stylized performances, self-representations, and the commodification of their own bodies as digital influencers, spokeswomen, entrepreneurs, and consumers. By grounding theoretical arguments in Black women's real experiences, and by taking seriously what they tell and show us, we can decolonize beauty studies to better understand the meaning of Black hair in the twenty-first century.

Researching Black Hair

This book focuses on the experiences of women of African descent and their in-person and online interactions with the natural hair community, as told to and observed by me over the course of six years. Between 2013 and 2018, I conducted 79 interviews with people who participate in natural hair movement spaces across four continents.[42] Then, from 2018 to 2021, I continued to read, watch, and observe as this evolving conversation found new manifestations, shapes, and platforms. Through interviews and observations across multiple field sites, I paint a detailed and nuanced portrait of the meanings of femininity, naturalness, and racial authenticity as they play out on and through Black women's bodies.

I met and recruited interviewees through local organizations for Black women, during my fieldwork at hair shows and in beauty salons, in online natural hair forums, and by referral. I had many hours-long conversations in their homes, neighborhoods, and communities. While I did not have the means to pay interviewees, I usually offered to purchase their coffee to thank them for sharing their time with me. I collected identifying information about my interviewees, which allowed me to schedule follow-up conversations when necessary and identify trends across demographics. I gathered personal histories about hairstyling choices, their experience of "going natural," and their re-flections about natural hair as a movement. I interviewed mostly lay *naturalistas*, or women for whom natural hair is not a part of their career, because they are the main participants in natural hair shows, the primary readers of natural hair blogs, and the intended audience for vlog reviews of products. I also spoke with people who manage, lead, and create spaces for natural hair communities; these organizers provided insight on the community aspect of the natural hair move-ment and articulated the objectives of the events they held. During interviews with natural hair organizers, I inquired about their po-litical commitments, intergroup relationships, organizational forms, movement trajectories, and labor demands. I asked business owners about their entrepreneurship histories, business plans, perspectives on beauty trends, product sourcing, industry networks, relationships with customers, and retail mediums. These interviews helped me to understand the changing modes and landscapes of ethnic entrepre-neurship and interethnic conflict within the beauty industry. I noted convergences and divergences in how and to what extent interviewees deployed movement terminology to construct meanings around natu-ral hair for Black women.

Several of the people that I spoke with kept in contact with me over the years, forwarding me articles of interest that they came across or written reflections of memories that surfaced after we spoke. I found that most were eager to talk about this topic, and our ongoing interac-tions demonstrated that many other people were also actively engaged in contemplating the significance of this new natural hair movement.

Instead of observing people in a single place, I attended dozens of natural hair shows, beauty industry conventions, and online spaces across four continents. Multi-sited ethnography acknowledges that people, connections, associations, and relationships may be substantially continuous even as they are spatially or organizationally noncontinu-ous,[43] and made sense for this project because the natural hair move-ment is global and interconnected by way of social media, transnational commerce, and internationally-touring natural hair gatherings. A community of beauty bloggers, natural hair organizers, small business entrepreneurs, and laywomen attend each other's events, traveling across town, across the country, and across national borders to share information and vend products. I frequently encountered natural hair influencers repeatedly at one another's events and as featured models on online natural hair forums. As I travelled internationally, I often relied on natural hair influencers in the United States to introduce me to their collaborators abroad.

Most of my research occurred at hair shows and beauty industry conventions. Natural hair events are ideal sites to conduct this research because they are spaces where organizers, bloggers, stylists, retailers, and lay consumers come together to interactively discuss and shape body politics in person. Some natural hair shows are small and intimate, attracting fifteen to twenty attendees in a neighborhood hair salon or restaurant. Other meetups are massive, with many vendors and tens of thousands of participants. The largest natural hair expos are held on an annual basis. Smaller meetups occur more frequently, at least twice a week in major cities and at about monthly in less-populated metropolitan areas. Ethnographic immersion allowed me to provide detailed descriptions of the cultural, social, and physical contexts that matter to natural hair culture.

The US-based data for this project came primarily from fieldwork in three cities: Atlanta, New York City, and Los Angeles. Atlanta, colloquially known as the "Black hair capital," hosts the largest Black beauty industry expos and the oldest natural hair shows, and so draws many aspiring entrepreneurs. Fieldwork in Atlanta allowed me to contextualize both natural hairstyles and the emergent natural hair movement's place within the Black haircare industry at large. I traveled to Atlanta four times to attend the 2014 and 2015 Taliah Waajid World Natural Hair Shows, as well as the 2015 and 2016 Bronner Bros. International Hair Shows. Each trip to Atlanta lasted around one week. During these visits, I took notes at workshops, expo spaces, and associated expo gatherings.

I also spent ten months in New York, where I attended natural hair workshops around the city and interviewed women of African descent in beauty shops. New York is a global city and enabled greater ethnic diversity in my sample. Its communities of African and Caribbean immigrant women allowed me to probe multiple local and diasporic meanings of Blackness and beauty. I also spent three years attending natural hair events around Los Angeles, my home during my doctoral program at the University of Southern California. Los Angeles's role as an entertainment hub provided easy access to high-profile vloggers and women who navigate what "looks" sell in the media marketplace, illuminating how tastemakers are currently constructing who and what is considered beautiful.

I explored the international dimensions of the natural hair movement through interviews with women in Spain, the Netherlands, France, South Africa, and Brazil, which expanded my understanding of how national racial regimes and histories influence the meanings of natural hair in these specific contexts. I further attended to questions of the global by spending two months in Cape Town and Johannesburg in 2016. Given the geographic and economic constraints of conducting qualitative research on a global phenomenon like the natural hair movement, I chose South Africa as a strategic site for two reasons: 1) the presence of a multiracial "Coloured" category provides a useful comparison to the US's "one-drop-rule" measure of Blackness, which illuminated the relationship between racial boundaries and local beauty ideals, and 2) South Africa, like most African countries, has a fraught relationship with a US- and Asian-dominated human hair and cosmetics industry, impacting Black and Coloured women's access to consumer products for natural hair. These two features allowed me to probe why and how natural hair has become a site for organizing for women of African descent in different cultural and economic contexts at the same historical moment. Having lived in South Africa for six months while I attended the University of Cape Town in college, I benefitted from prior relationships with sociologists, media studies scholars, feminist collectives, and communities of Black and Coloured South Africans who facilitated my research process overseas. Comparative global research revealed that racial politics and racial formation projects at the state and individual levels draw from internationally-circulating discourses across the Black Atlantic. While racial categories across the African diaspora differ, parallel experiences of European colonization, racial slavery, and white domination unite people of African descent in Europe, the Caribbean, the Americas, and West Africa in a common Black consciousness, understanding, and experience of race and racialization.[44] The Middle Passage was not a one-way or final moment of transfer of African peoples across the Atlantic. Africana people in the Americas, the Caribbean, Europe, and on the African continent have continued to communicate, finding inspiration in one another's art, politics, and experiences. For Black women, fashion and style have been important modes for facilitating and circulating global political exchange.[45]

My research also extended to social media platforms, because natural hair discourse is widely circulated, constructed, and disseminated on the internet. Online spaces have become another "level" where participants live their everyday lives.[46] Through an ecosystem of social networks, geographically-distant groups of women connect, converse, collaborate, purchase, and plan. My findings demonstrate that online interactions do more than overlap with face-to-face interactions; they are integral to business structures and the construction of community among geographically-distant groups of women of African descent. I immersed myself in many sites where natural hair is regularly discussed, including accounts on Facebook, Instagram, YouTube, and Tumblr. My interviewees frequently referenced social media destinations where they learn haircare techniques, identify local natural hair events, watch product reviews, and broadly engage with body politics. I noted their references and recorded observations in and of the online places that they suggested. I also recruited some interviewees from online natural hair forums.

This research is interested in understanding the experiences of women of African descent who are similarly positioned within intersecting race and gender hierarchies, capitalist structures, and who share a history or experience of living in places with legacies of white supremacist colonialism and slavery.[47] I am interested in what it is like to be a woman of African descent with natural hair, as well as the subjective experience of Blackness and womanhood in the context of contemporary culture. The focus of this book is on how Black women talk about hair *in their own terms*, rather than in comparison to Black men or white women, foregrounding how and whether Black women construct race, class, gender, and cultural hierarchies within spaces that celebrate natural hair. I asked my respondents to help me identify and refine who is welcome to participate in the natural hair movement's collective identity in an attempt to understand the contours of this ever-shifting global community.

As I reviewed my conversations and interactions, I sought to understand the ways in which my participants construct boundaries around an identity-based movement and respond to dominant beauty ideals, controlling images of Black womanhood, and an extended history of economic exclusion from the beauty industry and marketplace. By giving voice to the everyday experiences of women who are marginalized by race, gender, and often class, this study aims to illuminate the lived effects of power relations at the intersection of race and gender hierarchies in places with histories of slavery and European settler colonialism.

This book will take you on a journey of how naturalistas' embodied experiences and beauty practices became tied up with processes of politicization and organizing for social change. This tale, however, is as old as time (or really, as old as European colonialism and chattel slavery): the natural hair movement is just the most recent manifestation of Black women's ongoing struggles for bodily autonomy. The following chapter provides historical context of Black women's hairstyling, beauty cultures, and politics through the theoretical lens of racial formation. For centuries, politicizing beauty has enabled Africana women to imagine their lives and their bodies differently—despite patriarchal, economic, and racial domination. As dominant social justice strategies, theories for change, and understandings of racial uplift have shifted, so too have Black women's politics of style. So, let us return to the beginning. Let us be present for this homecoming. Let us see how, to borrow I.S. Jones's words, each curl became a war cry.

1

Hair Sankofa

A History of Black Hair Politics

Aunt Jemima's checkered headscarf, framing wide eyes and an even wider smile, on millions of kitchen shelves around the world. Kathleen Cleaver's defiant Afro, perched high and round, with a clenched fist to match. Venus Williams's bead-flanked braids and the outrage at their technicolor tumble onto the Australian Open tennis court. While beauty is often thought of as apolitical, or even counterpolitical, the ways that Black women's bodies have been styled, represented, talked about, and treated have never been minor nor inconsequential. Each of these moments in Black beauty also represent key projects of gendered racial (re)formation in our race- and gender-obsessed society.

Since bodies are also deeply symbolic of and affected by class and gender hierarchies, women across the African diaspora have often politicized beauty in their various fights for liberation, self-definition, and social change, dating back to the earliest eras of European colonization in Africa and the Americas. For Black women, beauty and styling practices are mutually informed by the pressures to avoid racism and violence, as well as by the pleasures of securing social, cultural, material, and aesthetic capital. As social conflicts evolved over time, and as communities reflected on their responses to those conflicts, Black folks continued to assign new and different meanings to race, gender, beauty, and style. This chapter theorizes the most pivotal eras in Black beauty history, examining moments in their historical context to determine shifting ideals of value, power, and beauty.

As the Ghanaian concept of Sankofa asserts, we can only understand our present if we understand what has come before. A history of

Black beauty activism is essential to understanding the gravity, shape, and meaning of this century's natural hair movement—one of the most recent ways Black women have used beauty to work and rework their place within racial, gender, and economic systems—because it reacts, remixes, and reconstitutes prior thinking about how to free Black people and Black bodies. Before we focus on the new natural hair movement, let us turn our gaze to the past.

Slavery, Colonization, and Racializing Hair Texture

The power arrangements contextualizing today's natural hair movement began to take shape when European explorers arrived in the Americas in 1492, the year that Spanish explorer Christopher Columbus first encountered the island now known as the Bahamas. By the mid-sixteenth century, Dutch, French, Spanish, British, and Portuguese pilgrims were claiming land in the Americas and Caribbean for themselves in a race for wealth and territory. As these colonizers settled in the "New World," they displaced, killed, and forced Indigenous peoples into indentured servitude alongside other Europeans, most of whom were English, Scottish, or Irish. After stopping in port cities like Cape Town and Durban, South Africa, English and Dutch colonizers also transported thousands of sub-Saharan Africans, East Indians, and Indonesians as indentured servants to the North and South Americas, as well as to Caribbean territories like Suriname, Trinidad and Tobago, Guyana, and Jamaica. Planters set up large estates for farming cash crops like fruits, vegetables, cotton, tobacco, and sugar, powered by enslaved people of African descent.[1] These interrelated systems of European colonization on the African continent and chattel slavery in the Americas and Caribbean first racialized culturally diverse sub-Saharan African peoples as a cohesive social category: Black. Since intricate hair-braiding styles and head adornments are traditional symbols of pride, spirituality, and clan status in most African cultures, denigrating enslaved Africans' hair was central to denying them their identity. One of the first acts of suppression

slave traders did was shave the heads of their captives, which symbolically revoked the enslaved people's sense of belonging to their tribe of
origin and ownership over their own body.[2] Slave traders also refused
enslaved people their given birth names, treating their human captives
like anonymous chattel cargo. Enslaved people were no longer Ashanti,
Igbo, Mende, Yoruba, or Mandingo—they were Negro, Black, enslaved,
inferior. As the demand for labor grew, Europeans increased their
slave-trading operations in West Africa.[3] By the nineteenth century,
an estimated twenty million Africans had been transported across the
Atlantic in bondage.[4] By the seventeenth century, indentured servitude
in the Americas had been largely replaced by a peculiar race-based system of slavery that constructed white supremacy against Black servitude.

Sociologists Michael Omi and Howard Winant's theory of racial formation defines race as "a concept which signifies and symbolizes social
conflicts and interests by referring to different types of human bodies."[5]
Race is not an essential or biological characteristic, but a socially constructed category of difference that determines a group's material, political, and social status.[6] Racialization, in turn, is the process by which
a ruling group justifies its position by asserting that the phenotypical
features of the oppressed groups—like Black peoples' coily and kinky
hair textures—express their essential and biological inferiority.[7] Those
in power further legitimate their societal privilege through racialized
political, religious, academic, and artistic representations and discourses
circulating at the macro level. Think: minstrel shows that depict Black
people as stupid, jolly workers in order to justify their fitness for servitude, or for a more modern example, discourses that describe Black
women as conniving "welfare queens" that take advantage of social
safety nets in order to justify limits on government assistance. To this
day, in regions where the slave trade dominated, white people remain in
power, and harmful racist stereotypes and social norms are maintained
by structures of white supremacy.[8] Current racial conflicts and social dynamics only make sense by acknowledging how this backdrop of slavery
and colonization have been central organizing forces in society.

Enslaved people often lacked the tools, the time, and the conditions to care for their hair with the herbal ointments, combs, and oils they used in their African homelands. Scalp diseases and lice were common; racist stigmas of Black hair as dirty and unhealthy are rooted here.[9] Enslaved men and women who worked in the fields usually wore rags on their heads to protect their skin from the sun, sweat, grime, and parasites.[10] Many also shaved their heads or braided their hair in small sections to keep it from matting.[11] Those who worked in closer proximity to whites as cooks, washerwomen, housekeepers, and nursemaids were more likely to imitate European hairstyles, either donning powdered wigs or neat, tight plaits to avoid the ire of their slaveholders, who judged one another based on the health and condition of the people they enslaved.[12] If enslaved people had a day off, it was usually Sunday to observe the Sabbath, so Sundays became days for spiritual renewal and self-care. Former slave Amos Lincoln recalled in an interview with the Federal Writer's Project years after emancipation, "All week they wear they hair all in a roll with cotton that they unfold from the cotton boll. Sunday come they come [comb] they hair fine. No grease on it. They want it nice and naturally curly."[13] Wash day, a day set apart for self-care through haircare, continues to be a spiritual ritual for many Black women.

Racial mixing was common among Africans, Europeans, East Indians, and Indigenous people in diversifying African port cities, as well as in colonies across the Americas and the Caribbean. British law in the sixteenth and early-seventeenth centuries decreed that a child inherited the racial status of their father, so any mixed-race child with a white father was free at birth. However, by the mid-1600s, most of those laws had been reversed in the American colonies. They were replaced by a new set of laws and norms that formed the basis of the "one-drop rule" of Black hypodescent in the United States. By reconstructing interracial mixing as a process of "Blackening" rather than "whitening," white slaveholders were able to increase their wealth by raping enslaved Black women to grow their enslaved population, and more broadly, these policies allowed white elites to stabilize an exclusive right to social authority.[14]

Anti-miscegenation laws encouraged people to scrutinize others for any African-looking phenotypical features and police the color line. Anyone with proven African ancestry was considered Black and at risk of enslavement. A commonsense understanding developed that Blackness, the inverse of white purity, contained a wide range of skin tones, ranging from very dark to very fair, and hair textures ranging from very coily to straight. As sociologist Kobena Mercer explains, "the pejorative precision of the salient expression, *nigger hair*, neatly spells out how, within racism's bipolar codification of human worth, Black people's hair has been historically devalued as the most visible stigmata of Blackness, second only to skin."[15] *Bad hair* is another term for nigger hair, the dichotomous opposite of *good hair*, a term used to describe Black hair closer to a Eurocentric standard of beauty—wavy, silky, smooth or loosely-curled. And, as Black hair historians Ayana D. Byrd and Lori L. Tharps point out, "more than one hundred years after the terms 'good' and 'bad' hair became part of the Black American lexicon, the concept endures."[16]

Distinctions between Blacks, mulattos, quadroons, and octoroons attempted to affirm and maintain the white-supremacist plantation economy and the racial caste system in the antebellum American South. Similar distinctions for interracial people developed in other parts of the world, like *coloured* in South Africa, *red* in Trinidad, and *parda, mulata,* and *morena* in Brazil. Colorism, the belief that those with visible proximity to whiteness are superior to those of the same racial group with darker skin, is a product of these hierarchical racial categorizations.[17] In other words, colorism refers to a system of stratification and differential treatment that privileges those with lighter complexions. Colorism and patriarchy work in tandem with texturism, or the idea that straight, long hair is more feminine, beautiful, and *good*.

Familial, spatial, and phenotypical proximity to whiteness shaped life for Black people in many ways. On plantations across the Caribbean, North America, and South America, mixed-race enslaved people with lighter skin and wavy or straight hair tended to enjoy an elevated status as domestic servants, observing and imitating white genteel etiquette.[18]

Darker-skinned enslaved people were often relegated to more strenuous physical labor in the fields. Some white slaveholders freed and sponsored the education of their mixed-race children, who formed much of the free Negro population in the American South and became the earliest Black professionals in the North. In some parts of Louisiana and South Carolina, free mixed-race communities served as a tertiary buffer class between more powerful whites and enslaved Blacks.[19] Since light skin and straight hair implied free status, some light-complexioned enslaved people passed as free or white to escape bondage. Many Black people internalized beliefs that straight hair was "good" and tightly coiled hair was "bad" and "nappy" because hair texture corresponded with privilege both on and off the plantation.[20] White slaveholders reinforced texturism by referring to Black people's hair as woolly, which further legitimized slavery by likening Black people to animals and excluding them from humanity. Discourses that curly hair textures were unruly, uncivilized, and closer to the earth implied that Black people were meant to toil the land and to be excluded from citizenship, thus reinforcing the logics of white supremacy and chattel slavery.

Racism, colorism, and texturism intersected with a patriarchal order to produce unique forms of oppression for Black women during slavery because systems of racism, capitalism, and patriarchy interlock and mutually reinforce each other.[21] While both women and men were exploited laborers under chattel slavery, enslaved Black women's sexual availability and reproductive capacity made them more susceptible to additional forms of objectification and commodification.[22] Many white male slaveholders and overseers forced sexual relationships with enslaved African women whom they viewed as their property. By the late-eighteenth century, it was commonplace for wealthy white men to openly keep Black mistresses.[23] Some mulatto, octoroon, and quadroon women were intentionally bred and sexually fetishized for their "exotic" beauty, and generated high bids at auctions where enslaved people were sold.[24] Mixed-race women's phenotypical and spatial proximity to whiteness made them particularly vulnerable to rape by white men and the wrath of their jealous wives.[25] In response, slaveholders' wives were known to shave off domestic servants' hair as a form of punishment, which operated as a gendered racial project to maintain white women's racial superiority over Black women in a patriarchal system that put them in competition for men's sexual attention. (But of course, Black and white women's "attention" from men took different forms and was experienced differently, since each group's social and political position vis-à-vis white men was dissimilar.) Rose Weitz reports that:

> In virtually every incident in which a slave was punished by having his or her head shaved, the punished slave was a woman with straight hair and the person who ordered the punishment was a white woman. By doing so, white women could reduce the threat these slaves posed to their marriages while punishing both the slaves and the white men who found them attractive.[26]

This disciplinary tactic demonstrates that both white women and Black women understood the significance, favor, risk, and access to power that long, loosely-textured hair and proximity to white beauty standards afforded.[27]

Black women's hair was taken up in a variety of other disciplinary gendered racial projects during slavery. In 1785, Spanish colonial governor of Louisiana Esteban Rodriguez Miró passed a sumptuary law mandating that Black women wear *tignons*, or handkerchief head wraps, to visibly mark themselves as belonging to the slave class and thus different from and inferior to whites, regardless of skin tone or free status.[28] The Tignon Laws also provided white men with a needed defense against the "lure" of mixed-race women's erotically "exotic" hair. By reinforcing the white patriarchal order, the Tignon Laws reflected the growing preoccupation with controlling women's sexuality, and asserted that women must compete with one another for men's attention, a challenge that further advanced the white beauty ideal. Sumptuary laws mandating that women of African descent identify and discipline themselves by wearing cloth coverings over their hair also governed those living in French, Dutch, and British colonies in the Caribbean through the late 1800s.[29]

Racial formation theory acknowledges that hegemonic ideologies about race and gender are not totally coercive, but are shaped through the consent or resistance of subordinated groups. Racialization, like all hegemonic practices, is not fixed, but responds to competing representations. Those with less privilege and who lack institutional power also influence and drive the content and results of racial projects. After all, as Omi and Winant argue, racial formation is a "continuing encounter between despotic and democratic practices, in which individuals and groups confronted by state power and entrenched privilege but not entirely limited by those obstacles make choices and locate themselves over and over in the constant racial 'reconstruction' of everyday life."[30] In other words, resistance efforts by marginalized groups participate in the process of racial formation by producing alternative discourses and applying pressure to the state and the economy. Institutions, in turn, respond to movements of resistance by shifting policies and definitions. New moments of racial formation are constantly unfolding.

Black women's reactions to the Tignon Laws exemplify this dynamic process of racial articulation and rearticulation. Many Afro-Creole women in Louisiana with economic means protested the spirit of the Tignon Laws by decorating their headscarves with jewels, ribbons, and feathers. Elaborately-adorned tignons ultimately became a defiant fashion statement for free women of color in eighteenth-century Louisiana and challenged the white supremacist patriarchal order. The ways in which Afro-Creole deployed style demonstrates how racial meanings are formed and reformed at the micro-level of the body and through the style choices that individual women make. While the reclamation of the tignon was an important symbolic act of bodily autonomy within the confines of a system of enslavement, tales of enslaved Black people in North and Central America using braiding patterns to relay secret messages to one another, as maps to direct each other to the North or to maroon communities, or as hiding places for seeds. These practices reveal how Black hair culture and hair styling have also been literally integral in some Black people's pursuits to free themselves from enslavement entirely.

While slaveholders in the United States continued to breed enslaved Black people in captivity after the slave trade was legally abolished in 1808, slaveholders in the Caribbean and South America continued to import additional laborers from Africa for decades later.[31] Perhaps because of this brutal replacement system, new arrivals to African communities in the Caribbean and South America continued to pass along more traditions from their homelands, enabling these communities to navigate the racist systems in unique ways. For example, enslaved women in the West Indies resisted sumptuary laws by communicating secret messages to one another through the architectural folds and positions of knots they manipulated into the material of their headscarves. These tignon codes were material links between Black Caribbean women and the traditions of their West African ancestors, who used intricate cloth-folding traditions to signify wealth, ethnicity, marital status, mourning, and reverence. Like Nigerian *geles* and Ghanaian *dukus* from across the Atlantic, Caribbean women's head wraps were notoriously dramatic. Historian Beverly Lemire writes that Black women's "apparent lack of deference to the disciplinary intent of the law irked settlers and some visitors who identified African Caribbean women as a source of social corruption."[32] Minority cultures of resistance, like these, routinely become sites where political contradictions are resolved, history is remembered, and alternatives are imagined.[33]

After the United States abolished slavery in 1865, some Black women in the United States continued to wear head wraps creatively, but the style ultimately became associated with servitude and homeliness. Wearing headscarves in public further fell out of favor among early-twentieth-century Black American communities following the mass production of mammy images like Aunt Jemima wearing a checkered hair tie. In contrast, Afro-Surinamese women elders have carried on head wrapping traditions through time, to the present, and through space, as they migrated in large numbers to form vibrant Africana communities in the Netherlands in the 1970s and 1980s. In hopes of shoring up economic opportunity, these women migrated to the Netherlands after being given the option to choose between Dutch and Surinamese citizenship in the lead up to Suriname's independence from the Netherlands in 1975. During the annual Keti Koti ("Breaking the Chains") festival in Amsterdam, which commemorates the abolition of slavery in former Dutch colonies, Surinamese and Antillean women march through the city proudly donning bright and towering head wraps as symbols of their resilient heritage and enduring connection to their culture and homeland across the Atlantic.

Styling Segregation and Respectability Politics

By the end of the Reconstruction period in the late 1800s, the rise of Jim Crow segregation enforced a two-tier racial system in the United States that subordinated all non-whites to whites. Black folks were subject to de facto and de jure racial discrimination in the job market, the electoral process, the school system, public spaces, and more.

White-owned companies dominated the Black haircare industry in the late 1800s, and their marketing messages commonly reinforced white supremacy and Black inferiority. A typical advertisement read: "Race men and women may easily have straight, soft, long hair by simply applying Plough's Hair Dressing and in a short time all your kinky, snarly, ugly hair becomes soft, silky, smooth . . ."[34] White legislators and physicians contributed to this white supremacist racial project by depicting Blacks as disease carriers and their barbershops as disease-ridden.[35] At the turn of the century, mainstream newspapers increasingly represented Black masculinity as violent through myths that white women were at high risk for sexual assault by Black men. Black male hairdressers' close bodily contact with whites became increasingly viewed as suspect and dangerous.[36] Stereotypes of Black men as criminally-hypersexual maintained white supremacy and perceptions of Black powerlessness, and incited extralegal lynch mobs across the American South. The impact these prejudices had on Black workers' access to employment at white-owned salons narrowed an established pathway for Black men's entry into the middle class. Barbering and salon service work progressively became segregated by race, ultimately becoming what Adia Harvey Wingfield terms a "racial enclave economy."[37]

At the same time, racial segregation also allowed beauty culture to become a critical avenue for Black women's upward mobility. Black beauty educators (or "culturists," as they called themselves) established cosmetology training institutes that offered Black women a rare opportunity to escape field labor, factory work, and domestic service. Beauty culturists Marjorie Stewart Joyner and J. H. Jemison famously taught thousands of Black women valuable business and trade skills, ushering many Black families into middle-class stability.[38] Joyner trained Madam C. J. Walker, who eventually became the first self-made woman millionaire in the United States. Walker lifted tens of thousands more Black American women out of poverty by training them to become independent door-to-door sales agents for her beauty products, in addition to her various philanthropic endeavors.[39] Eventually, in the postbellum, pre-Civil Rights era, ninety-five percent of working Black women who owned property were either hairdressers, washerwomen, or seamstresses.[40]

White elites responded to Black women's new opportunities in the beauty industry with repression. Lawmakers in Georgia imposed targeted taxes on Black hairdressing establishments, blaming the shortage of Black field labor on Black women's newfound opportunities in beauty culture.[41] To protect themselves, Walker, Joyner, Jemison, and others formed the National Beauty Culturists League (NBCL), which aimed to improve training standards and earnings within the cosmetology industry and collectively lobby for their interests. The NBCL endeavored to present Black women as civically responsible, self-sufficient, and enterprising without abandoning individual workers to racist and sexist legal and corporate systems.[42] Attracting thousands of entrepreneurs and practitioners, beauty shops became a near "depression-proof" enterprise for Black American women during the Great Depression.[43]

Beauty shop owner or hairstylist was the most autonomous occupation open to Black women during the Jim Crow era. Black beauty shops were also the most lucrative industry wherein all aspects—from education and service to atmosphere and consumption—were run by Black women.[44] Black beauticians challenged ideas that the business world and public sector should be male-only spaces. In addition, Black beauticians reclaimed the aspects of womanhood denied them during slavery.[45] During the Civil Rights Movement, Black beauty salons were one of few establishments that escaped white oversight. Unlike churches, salons were gendered spaces where Black women could foreground intersecting race and gender issues.[46] Many beauty shop owners used their salons to raise political consciousness among their clientele and to fight deprecating depictions of Black women in mainstream media.[47] Black beauticians also widely participated in the Black women's club movement and in racial justice organizations like the National Association for the Advancement of Colored People (NAACP) and Marcus Garvey's Universal Negro Improvement Association (UNIA).[48] Tiffany M. Gill explains, "the hair-care industry in general and the Black beauty parlor in particular should be examined as an important, albeit unique, institution in the Black community, a space that was once public and private, where the matrix of beauty, business, and politics allowed Black women to actively confront issues of their day."[49]

When Black women entered professional positions in increasing numbers post-World War II, many chose to straighten their hair for work, because head wraps and curly hair had long been taken up by the media and the state as symbolic of Black women's inferiority. Like Black clubwomen of the same period, beauty culturists promoted respectability as a pathway to acceptance by whites, and ultimately invented technologies to "press" or thermally straighten coiled hair.[50] In other words, they believed that Black women would be better off by emphasizing how they are culturally and morally similar to whites to gain their respect and acceptance.[51] Straight hair was considered neat and professional, so straightened hair successfully facilitated some white employers' tolerance of Black women's presence in the workplace. By deemphasizing physical differences between Blacks and whites, thermally straightened hair accentuated Black women's willingness to adhere to mainstream feminine beauty and professional norms. As many Black feminists have pointed out, in a global society where Black women fit at the bottom of race, gender, and often class hierarchies, adherence to white ideologies about beauty often improve Black women's opportunities for upward mobility via access to employment, social networks, and romantic relationships.[52] Historian Julia Kirk Blackwelder explains, "In the segregation era carefully groomed hair and immaculate dress armed women against the arrows of racial insults. Beauticians thus played a role in undermining Jim Crow and styling its defeat."[53] Even though straightened hair enabled many Black American women to reclaim the self-respect and dignity that whites systematically denied them, respectability politics also forced restrictive notions of femininity on Black women who were burdened with the responsibility to represent the race.[54]

During Jim Crow, Black men experienced their own conflicts around respectability and assimilation. The slicked back conk look—achieved through heavy pomades and chemical relaxers—came into style among young African American and Latino zoot-suiters in the 1930s and 1940s. In the 1950s, James Brown and Little Richard's slick, glistening hairdos epitomized cool. When the political climate changed in the latter half of the decade, the conk became seen as a shameful act of assimilation for those in the Black movement community. Perhaps the most iconic account and analysis of the conk appears in Malcolm X's 1964 autobiography. In the text, Malcolm X remembers admiring his reflection in the mirror after his friend Shorty assisted him in his first painfully traumatic application of lye relaxer to his scalp. He admits that his increased proximity to whiteness made him fall in love with his new image. In retrospect, Malcolm X describes this moment as his "first really big step toward degradation."[55] He goes on to lament, "I had joined that multitude of Negro men and women in America who are brainwashed into believing that the Black people are 'inferior'—and the white people 'superior'—that they will even violate and mutilate their God-created bodies to try to look 'pretty' by white standards."[56] Malcolm X came to eschew assimilationist rationales for hair straightening, asserting that wealthy Negroes "ought to know better" and praising celebrities like Sidney Portier for fighting through and against white standards of desirability to achieve success and acclaim in Hollywood.[57] Relaxers were never as widely adopted among Black men as they were among Black women, and they went out of fashion almost entirely for Black men by the 1960s.

Hair texture was also taken up in segregationist institutional policies and, in turn, a politics of respectability across the Atlantic. Under South Africa's apartheid rule, which lasted from 1948 to 1991, "bodies [were] signifiers of status, power, and worth in a hierarchy that privileged whiteness (as both a biological and social condition) at its apex."[58] The government classified its population into four categories: white, Coloured, Indian, and Black. The white minority controlled the government, land, and economy. One way that people strived for political, social, and economic power was by petitioning the government to reclassify their legal racial category as white. The appeal boards for reclassification scrutinized petitioners' phenotypical racial markers, like hair texture, cheekbones, and even the color of one's genitalia.[59] The most notorious method that the apartheid state used to determine "non-white" from "white" was the pencil test. If the petitioner's hair texture was straight enough for a pencil to fall out, he or she was more likely to be granted an official racial status adjustment. If the pencil remained instead of slipping out, the person's hair was considered too curly to belong to a white person. Thus, the texture of one's hair could determine whether they could marry their lover, attend university, or access adequate health care. In some cases, boards called upon barbers to testify about a petitioner's true hair texture, as people used hot combs and chemical relaxers to undermine the test. Importantly, no one was ever reclassified from Black to white or vice versa during apartheid, so hair texture was a critical factor for assimilating into elite society reserved only for Coloured and Indian South Africans, an opportunity not afforded Black South Africans. Apartheid rule left a lasting impression on cultural standards for corporate professionalism in South Africa that influence workers and students of all backgrounds, especially since whites still own a disproportionate amount of the country's land and capital. Hair straightening remains essential to many people of color in their quests for social and economic mobility. For Black women especially, relaxers remain a popular service in Black salons and in Black beauty culture as a sign of and reward for economic security.

Segregation resulted in both intra-racial solidarity and disparity in Black America. Hair straightening was not just a strategy for navigating white spaces; colorism and respectability politics contributed to the overrepresentation of Blacks with lighter skin and straighter hair in the Black American elite and in the popular press throughout the twentieth century.[60] Many light-complexioned African Americans used their privileges to advocate for Black issues, while others internalized their proximity to white supremacy. Elite Black clubs, fraternities, churches, and schools institutionalized colorism through paper bag and comb tests that excluded Black people with skin too dark or hair too "kinky."[61] Actresses Dorothy Dandridge and Lena Horne were the suitable faces of Black beauty. Until the 1960s, beauty pageants at Historically Black Colleges and Universities (HBCUs) almost exclusively recruited and crowned light-skinned women with long hair.[62] The interaction between class privilege and white beauty ideals manifested in Black idioms like *nappy hair* and *hair grades* that hierarchized intra-racial phenotypical differences among Black people, particularly Black women.[63] Similarly, Kia Caldwell finds that, in Brazil, good hair versus bad hair distinctions express a culture of white desirability and a fear of Black contamination, despite the country's public image as a racial democracy after slavery was abolished in 1888.[64]

Black activists, academics, families, ministers, and reporters consistently contested dominant ideas that straight hair was desirable, insisting that curly hair be seen as "good."[65] For instance, Booker T. Washington banned beauty culturists from teaching at Tuskegee Institute, a Black college he founded to provide Black people with practical skills training. At his National Negro Business League convention, Washington also banned beauty culturists from presenting.[66] Scholar W. E. B. Du Bois and activist Marcus Garvey were likewise critical of relaxers and skin-bleaching practices. Hair straightening to assimilate into the predominantly white professional workforce exemplified what Du Bois termed the double consciousness that African Americans develop to survive white supremacy. In his observations, Black Americans are "a sort of seventh son, born with a veil, and gifted with second-sight in this American world" because they are intimately familiar with the American ideal even as they are excluded from it based on their race.[67]

Against critiques of hair straightening, beauty culturists then—like many beauty theorists since—pointed to the simultaneous effects of class, culture, and subjectivity on Black women's beauty practices during Jim Crow. To sell their straightening products, Black beauty entrepreneurs deployed discourses about good grooming, health, and economic mobility in advertisements to avoid implying that curly hair textures were essentially inferior.[68] Maxine Leeds Craig argues that for many Black women in the early and mid-twentieth century, straight hair was more about "looking like a lady" than it was about "looking white."[69] Writers Ayana Byrd and Lori Tharps similarly point out that hair straightening was also a matter of appearing less "country" and more "cosmopolitan" during the Great Migration of Black Americans from the rural South to cities like Chicago, Detroit, St. Louis, Philadelphia, and New York.[70] In addition, beauty consumerism was on the rise for women of all races during the mid-twentieth century. It was common for both Black and white women with excess income to take weekly trips to the hair salon and process their hair.[71]

Black Is Beautiful, Soul Style, and the Aesthetics of Rebellion

During the 1960s and 1970s, a new aesthetics of rebellion took hold. In the United States, the Black Power Movement loudly and proudly challenged the internalization and institutionalization of colorism and texturism in society. Activists condemned the dominant assimilationist rationales of the early twentieth century, instead emphasizing that "for Black people to adopt *their* methods of relieving *our* oppression is ludicrous."[72] Maxine Leeds Craig explains, "for members of the Black movement community, one of the consequences of personal transformation was the politicization of their bodies and behavior that was formerly considered private."[73] Not straightening one's hair, favoring dark skin, and choosing lovers of color were all part of this line of thought. "Black is beautiful," the slogan went. James Brown's anthem "Say It Loud—I'm Black and I'm Proud" filled the airwaves, and magazines *Essence*, *Ebony*, and *Jet* portrayed Black women with Afros as hip, glamorous, and fashion-forward. Wearing round, picked-out Afros, also referred to as "naturals," became symbolic of resistant Black beauty. Corliss, a retired economist and college administrator I interviewed about her relationship to her hair, reflected on the shift from assimilationist to Afrocentric racial uplift strategies during our conversation:

Well, there was a Black Power movement going on then . . . You know, people started seeing themselves differently. You know, with the hair straight down like white people it's like copying white people . . . "I'm Black and I'm proud" got to be a popular saying, then people didn't want to copy white people's hair so much anymore. So, there was a wholesale shift from chemically processed hair to Afro.

This shift often put Black baby boomers in conflict with their parents of the "traditionalist" generation. Corliss told me:

Our parents were *not* into the Afros. They thought it was rebellious and kind of wild-like. And they were more conformist to the predominant culture. But still very proud of their Blackness but they didn't want to risk offending white people with outward appearance and being judged before people get to know us inwardly.

The Afro was definitely not an understated style. Its size and shape required that it be worn proudly like a crown, with one's head high and back upright. This requisite dignified posture was itself defiant in the face of hegemonic racist associations that tied Blackness to inferiority and shame.[74]

Black-owned companies did not shy away from politicizing the Afro to sell products and services.[75] Black business owners considered making a profit and supporting images of Black Power to be complementary goals that concurrently redistributed Black aesthetic and material power.[76] As Tanisha Ford explains, this "re-aestheticization of Blackness . . . created new value and political power for the Black body."[77]

In the United States, "Black Is Beautiful" was a racial project where "hair was shaped by a broader Black reconceptualization of American Black identity as an ethnic identity with cultural connections to Africa."[78] Afros were also adopted by the Black Power movement community in Great Britain, many of whom were similarly coming to identify as Afro-Caribbean.[79] Around this same time, Rastafarianism increased in visibility and militancy in Jamaica. Rastafarian loc'ed hairstyles are based in biblical doctrines that restrict the cutting of hair. By embracing the natural material qualities of coily African hair, locs are an embodied portrayal of the Rastafarian belief that the "Promised Land" of Zion is in Ethiopia. Like the Afro, locs invoked nature to portray an Afrocentric political, aesthetic, and ethnic affiliation with a mythical African homeland.[80] For movement communities across the Black Atlantic, "natural" hairstyles were part of a counterhegemonic nation-building project to redefine people of the diaspora as ethnically African rather than Negro.[81] This unified African homeland is more imagined than real, since neither the Afro nor locs refer to any existing West African cultural hairstyling practices. As Angeline Morrison argues, the Afro signified "the Africa of the imagination, a homeland that is on the bodies and in the hearts and minds of diaspora people."[82] Sociologist Kobena Mercer further points out that in African cultures, hair is more likely to be braided, plaited, or wrapped than to be left to grow "naturally," though Afros and locs became fashionable among West African women as media representations of celebrities like Bob Marley, Nina Simone, and Miriam Makeba circulated through the Black Atlantic.[83] In increasingly cosmopolitan cities like Accra and Lagos, Afros referenced these metropolitan images of Blackness rather than traditional cultural practices or a resistant political identity.[84] However, it is important to note that Black Power and Pan-Africanist movements across the Black Atlantic *did*, in fact, identify and communicate with activists in decolonial movements on the African continent, with whom they shared an anti-imperialist worldview. Tanisha Ford argues that Afros were part of a global "soul style" that connected the Black Consciousness Movement in South Africa to the Black Power movements in Great Britain and the United States.[85]

Activists Angela Davis, Kathleen Cleaver, Huey Newton, and Jesse Jackson became global cultural figures not just because of their anti-racist politics, but also because of their hair. Both men and women in the Black movement community considered wearing an Afro a symbol of Black pride and liberation, which simultaneously undermined binary, oppositional gender norms and white-supremacist aesthetics. Afros meant more for Black women, however, because short coily hair did not conform to norms for "doing" heterosexual womanhood appropriately. As Robin Kelley explains of the 1970s Afro, "For Black women, more so than Black men, going 'natural' was not just a valorization of Blackness or Africanness, but a direct rejection of a conception of female beauty that many Black men themselves had upheld."[86] This resulted in conflicting intra-racial hierarchies and dilemmas for Black women. Some heterosexual Black men considered women with Afros to be outside the bounds of feminine desirability, while others judged Black women's political commitments based on their ability to achieve a culturally relative but still exclusionary beauty ideal. An intersectional analysis of the 1970s

Afro reveals its limited potential as a radical racial formation project at the same time that gender norms, heteronormativity, and fallacies of racial purity challenged many Black women's ability to embody "Black Is Beautiful" in ways that felt safe and empowering.[87]

The media and political representations of Angela Davis's Afro were especially influential to how natural hairstyles were interpreted when worn by Black women. When the United States Federal Bureau of Investigations (FBI) pursued and prosecuted the scholar-activist in 1970 under charges of alleged kidnapping, murder, and conspiracy, the government and press circulated photographs taken by activists, reporters, and undercover police that highlighted her "rebellious" Afro. When she was added to the FBI Ten Most Wanted Fugitives list, she went into hiding for two months. During and after this period, Davis estimates that "hundreds, perhaps even thousands, of Afro-wearing Black women were accosted, harassed, and arrested."[88] The Afro-wearing Black woman's association with Davis's alleged criminality, political extremism, and deviance persists to this day—a topic I will discuss in detail in Chapters 3 and 6.

Persistent racism, including the Afro's association with deviant behavior, meant that embodying "Black is Beautiful" was always a risky choice. Most Black women continued to straighten their hair through the 1960s and 1970s despite powerful attempts by activists, Black media, and artists to redefine natural hair as fashionable and political.[89] For women who came of age during the 1970s, political identity, fashion trends, family pressures, workplace demands, and personal preferences mutually shaped individual style. For example, Corliss (62, North Carolina) had grown up having her hair lovingly straightened in her neighbor's kitchen with a hot comb heated by the stove. She remembers relishing in the positive attention her Shirley Temple curls attracted at school. A lifetime of socialization meant that an understanding of straight hair as "good hair" was hard to break. As college students, Corliss and her friends' hairstyling choices were also strongly shaped by their class aspirations,

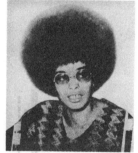

WANTED BY THE FBI

INTERSTATE FLIGHT - MURDER, KIDNAPING
ANGELA YVONNE DAVIS

FBI No. 867,615 G

Photograph taken 1969   Photograph taken 1970

Alias: "Tamu"

DESCRIPTION

Age:	26,	**Eyes:**	Brown
Height:	5'8"	**Complexion:**	Light brown
Weight:	145 pounds	**Race:**	Negro
Build:	Slender	**Nationality:**	American
Hair:	Black		
Occupation:	Teacher		
Scars and Marks:	Small scars on both knees		

Fingerprint Classification:

CAUTION

ANGELA DAVIS IS WANTED ON KIDNAPING AND MURDER CHARGES GROWING OUT OF AN ABDUCTION AND SHOOTING IN MARIN COUNTY, CALIFORNIA, ON AUGUST 7, 1970. SHE ALLEGEDLY HAS PURCHASED SEVERAL GUNS IN THE PAST. CONSIDER POSSIBLY ARMED AND DANGEROUS.

A Federal warrant was issued on August 15, 1970, at San Francisco, California, charging Davis with unlawful interstate flight to avoid prosecution for murder and kidnaping (Title 18, U. S. Code, Section 1073).

IF YOU HAVE ANY INFORMATION CONCERNING THIS PERSON, PLEASE NOTIFY ME OR CONTACT YOUR LOCAL FBI OFFICE. TELEPHONE NUMBERS AND ADDRESSES OF ALL FBI OFFICES LISTED ON BACK.

DIRECTOR
FEDERAL BUREAU OF INVESTIGATION
UNITED STATES DEPARTMENT OF JUSTICE
WASHINGTON, D. C. 20535
TELEPHONE, NATIONAL 8-7117

Entered NCIC
Wanted Flyer 457
August 18, 1970

FIGURE 1.1. FBI Wanted poster for Black Panther Party member Angela Davis (1970). Courtesy of the Smithsonian National Museum of African American History and Culture.

which often demanded that they adhere to a politics of respectability. Corliss further explained:

> Of my friends, the ones who were more studious and everything, they tended to have the chemically processed hair or they got their hair straightened with a hot comb. They kept with the straight hair and a little bit of Afrocentric jewelry instead of Afrocentric attire to kind of straddle both worlds, you know? I think the more studious friends were thinking, "I'm going the route that's going to get me as far as I can go in life, so, that means I gotta walk a fine line and not offend the white people but still get along with the Black people." So yeah. My friends were ambitious.

Corliss's friends' decisions to straighten their hair were acts of what Du Bois called double consciousness, anticipating that white gatekeepers would react negatively to Afrocentric style in the workplace. Ironically, artifice enabled some Black women to adopt "natural" hairstyles during this time. Corliss opted for a curly Afro wig so that she could easily transition between "soul style," which was popular at her Historically Black College, and white aesthetic standards for professionalism at her internships. Black women have always been resilient, finding creative ways to negotiate competing pressures and ideological systems to attain what they desire. Their everyday style practices subverted the logic of binary oppositionality between the "cultured" West and a traditionally "natural" Africa, which, Mercer points out, the Black Power Movement's liberation ideology also relied upon.[90]

The backlash against the Afro was swift. Physicians argued that Afros fostered unhealthy grooming habits, and Black beauticians pushed relaxers to encourage clients to purchase more-frequent services.[91] The mainstream media also downplayed the Afro's political dimensions and marketed the style as a fashionable trend.[92] This ultimately served to reduce the style's revolutionary Black Nationalist symbolism.[93] Angela Davis reflected on the lasting effects of her own Afro's commodification decades later: "It is humiliating because it reduces a politics of liberation to a politics of fashion; it is humbling because such encounters with the younger generation demonstrate the fragility and mutability of historical images, particularly those associated with African American history."[94] Afro wigs ultimately became kitschy nostalgia. And ironically, after centuries of denigrating curly hair textures and West African hairstyles, braids gained widespread popularity among white women when Bo Derek wore her hair in beaded cornrows in the 1980 movie *10*. Derek received credit for the style, angering many Black women who considered this cultural appropriation.[95] While men and women of the Black movement community had worn cornrows and Afros to express a diasporic collective identity in the previous decade, white women were donning the styles to express their individuality and eccentricity.

Also during the 1970s, Black American beauty culturists, including designers, models, and hairstylists in the entertainment industry, continued to circulate a "respectable" Black aesthetic in elite overseas markets.[96] They traveled to France, Italy, and England to capitalize on a greater acceptance of African Americans outside of the United States as a way grow their businesses and gain legitimacy. Bethann Hardison, Beverly Johnson, Pat Cleveland, and Naomi Sims became international supermodels. As they traveled, they established themselves as leading experts on Black beauty and haircare. Rather than advancing Black Nationalist or separatist ideologies, these beauty culturists sought to widen popular understandings of Western citizenship. Becoming "global ambassadors for American consumer capitalism," they saw themselves as uplifting the race by disseminating images of Black people as respectable, upwardly mobile, fashionable, and characteristically *American* during the Cold War era.[97] As they traveled across the Black Atlantic, beauty culturists expanded the image of American beauty in the global public consciousness to include dark skin, resisting sexist and racist tropes about Black women as animalistic, uncouth, and uncool.[98] By the end of the decade, the Afro was just as much about fashion, trendiness, and looking hip as it was about Black Power. This was the beginning of what sociologist Ashley Mears calls the "high-end ethnic aesthetic" in her ethnography of the fashion industry.[99]

Black Hair in the '80s, '90s, and 'oos

Hip-hop culture popularized new forms of fashion, dance, and music in the 1980s and 1990s, providing alternative representations of Black beauty and style that challenged Eurocentric beauty norms, especially for young people. Rappers and emcees gave voice to experiences of social and economic exclusion while creating alternative avenues for fame, wealth, and acclaim.[100] Hip-hop culture quickly spread throughout the world to become a powerfully influential form of postcolonial resistance across the Black Atlantic. Hip-hop fashion rejected white, middle-class styling norms.[101] Masculine style included baggy clothes, stocking caps, tattoos, and large jewelry. Timothy J. Brown explains the gendered effects of hip-hop style for Black men: "The *stylin* and *profiling* associated with a hip-hop Black masculinity is perpetuated in videos, films, entertainment, and athletics as a way to demonstrate an oppositional identity that is reified as a sign of a strong Black man."[102] The Philly fade was a popular hairstyle among rappers, emcees, deejays, and break dancers, featuring short hair on the sides of the head and a high flat top. Some people embellished their haircuts by etching elaborate designs and logos into their scalps.

Women and girls of the hip-hop generation often donned long extension braids, platinum blonde weaves, elaborate cornrows, and ornate updos crafted with wire, synthetic hair, and gel. Hip-hop style was imaginative, distinctly Black, proudly working class, and perhaps most identifiable by the defining look in the cult classic film *B.A.P.S.* (1997), starring a young Halle Berry. Many hip-hop hairstyles made use of the material qualities and sculptural potential of coily hair, as well as new technologies of artifice.[103] Black queer femmes were central innovators in this more playful, creative, and colorful Black hair and beauty landscape. As a result, Black politics of style became less and less binary, as

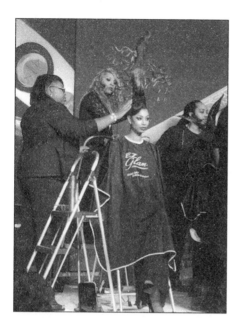

FIGURE 1.2. Hairstylist with model at a Black beauty show. Author's photo.

symbolized in drag queen RuPaul's hit single "Back to My Roots" (1992). RuPaul loudly proclaims, "Black hair is a revolution," donning a rotating display of blonde faux locs, cascading curls, and interlocking braided updos. In kitchens, bars, night clubs, and beauty shops, Black stylists found ways to make hairpieces defy gravity, spin, and light up. The best beauticians gained notoriety for their work by competing in runway competitions at Black beauty industry expositions. Black hair shows remain a rare space for Black stylists to showcase the craft and creativity of a distinctively Black style.

In the late 1990s and 2000s, artists Erykah Badu, Alicia Keys, Lauryn Hill, Jill Scott, and India Arie popularized towering head wraps, locs, braided extensions, and natural hair for a new generation. Arie's hit single "I Am Not My Hair" (2006) celebrated Black people's diverse and sometimes paradoxical hairstyling practices, as influenced by respectability politics, state surveillance, hip-hop culture, Afrocentricity, illness, and individual creativity alike. Just as the neo-soul genre repackaged Black music traditions like jazz, hip-hop, and R&B, these artists' hairstyles paid tribute to a rich history of Black hair culture and a Black feminist politics of resistance. Head wraps were new and unfamiliar to many outside the African diasporic community, but they quickly became a symbol of 1990s multiculturalism—a political philosophy encouraging diverse ethnic groups to collaborate with one another while retaining their distinctive identities. On an iconic episode of *Sesame Street* (1997), Erykah Badu used her colorful, plaid head wrap to teach children about tolerance and cross-cultural friendship. On the hit show *Moesha* (1996–2001) and in the made-for-TV movie *Cinderella* (1997), singer-actress Brandy made braids the "girl next door" style of choice for Black teenagers around the world.

Though a distinctively Black style flourished in the arts, debates about Black style in sports and the corporate world reminded the public that hip-hop hair was still exotic, risky, and marginal. When tennis stars Venus and Serena Williams entered the elite tennis scene with bold patterned outfits and technicolor hair, they were hit with scandal after scandal ignited by the media, fans, and pro tennis officials' responses to their "urban" fashion and hairstyling choices. Most memorably, Venus Williams was warned and penalized at the 1999 Australian Open because beads fell off her braids and onto the court. The referee argued the beads caused a "disturbance" to her opponent Lindsay Davenport. Williams ultimately lost the game. Until then, the rule had only been applied when larger garments like hats fell onto the court. Many saw the referee's call as a way of protecting the predominantly white and wealthy aesthetics in professional tennis culture. Black male celebrities also negotiated stereotypes that hip-hop style signified toxic Black masculinity and criminality. In the late '90s and early 'oos, Allen Iverson, with his cornrow braids, tattoos, baggy clothes, and use of African American Vernacular English (AAVE), became the NBA's most notorious player for his refusal to adopt white middle-class cultural norms after becoming wealthy. Brown summarizes, "For African American males such as Iverson who attempt to construct identities outside of the acceptable boundaries of dominant culture, their struggle for self-definition reflects the larger cultural clash between white society's middle-class values and Black masculinity from a hip-hop perspective."[104]

Likewise, as more Black women made cracks in the glass ceiling in the workplace, the conditions of inclusion in the corporate world often required adherence to Eurocentric beauty norms coded into professional standards. Employers and state institutions in South Africa, the Americas, and Western Europe adopted "color-blind" approaches to social problems that saw race-conscious policies reframed away from explicitly racist language while continuing to systematically perpetuate cultural forms of prejudice.[105] Color-blind language tends to shelter institutions from accusations of racial discrimination because race is often not mentioned, even if it is implicitly inscribed. For example, discriminatory and white-centered grooming policies in schools, the military, and the workplace institutionalize gendered racism, discouraging or explicitly preventing individuals from wearing culturally Black hairstyles like Afros, braids, and locs. Without mentioning race, such rules are still based in white, middle-class standards and disproportionately affect Black women because they are more likely than men to be judged by their appearance and to wear their hair long. Such policies become roadblocks constraining Black women's upward mobility via access to employment, social networks, and educational institutions.[106] As sociologist and Black feminist scholar Patricia Hill Collins explains, "where segregation used to keep Black women out of the classroom and boardroom, surveillance now becomes an important mechanism of control."[107] Many Black women were told or intuited that they needed to relax their hair to keep their jobs through grooming policies that defined professional hair as sleek, implying that curly hair is inherently unkempt. Audre Lorde points out that "in order to survive, those of us for whom oppression is as American as apple pie have always had to be watchers, to become familiar with the language of the oppressor, even sometimes adopting them for some illusion of protection."[108]

Those Black women who resisted conformity found themselves unprotected in a legal system that could only recognize one identity—race or gender—at a time. In legal cases where Black women plaintiffs argued they were racially discriminated against by employers for wearing natural or braided hairstyles, an unarticulated baseline of feminine whiteness and masculine Blackness made Black women's claims unintelligible.[109] These cases took center stage in the 1980s and 1990s. Consider the most famous of these incidents: *Rogers v. American Airlines*. In 1981, Renee Rogers sued her employer, American Airlines, for racial discrimination after she was fired for wearing cornrows to her job as a desk ticket agent. Rogers lost her appeal at the Federal District Court of New York because the judge argued that Rogers's hairstyle was influenced by Bo Derek's cornrows in the film *10* rather than her Black cultural heritage.[110] The decision implicitly asserted that white women's perception of cornrows as fashion determines how everyone else derives meaning from the style. It also ignored the ways in which hair is simultaneously gendered, racially constitutive, and culturally expressive.

Even as corporate forces policed their Black workers' bodies, they also began to recognize the profitability of Black hair. White-owned beauty companies reacknowledged Black women as profitable potential consumers and entered the "ethnic" haircare market in force in the 1980s and 1990s. While the Black haircare market had served as an ethic enclave economy for Black entrepreneurs for almost a century, by the mid-1980s most Black-owned beauty product manufacturers in the United States had been bought out by white-owned businesses. Historian Juliet E. K. Walker points out the role of racial discrimination in Black Americans' economic struggles: "If Black financial achievements seem inconsequential, it is not that Blacks have failed to save, but that capital available has been unconscionably circumscribed by race."[111] For much of the history of the United States, government policies exclusively subsidized and established contract agreements with white-owned companies, deliberately, systematically, and institutionally hindering Black business growth.[112] The usurpation of Black beauty businesses was largely facilitated by these sorts of racially-discriminatory regulatory and financial lending practices. For example, in 1975, the Federal Trade Commission

(FTC) ordered Johnson Products, the first Black-owned company to be listed on the American Stock Exchange, to add a health risk warning label to their Ultra Sheen relaxer. The FTC did not enforce the same policy against Johnson Products's largest competitor, white-owned Revlon, which used the same ingredients but advertised themselves as "better and safer."[113] Johnson Products sued the FTC and won twenty-two months later, but they never recovered from the incident and lost their market share to Revlon. In an infamous news article, Revlon executive Irving Bottner predicted that Black-owned cosmetics companies would eventually disappear altogether, stating that "they'll all be sold to White companies."[114] Since the haircare industry is at the center of many important Black economic milestones, losing racial ownership within it was fraught with emotional, moral, and material stakes. Bottner's remark incited Jesse Jackson and his Operation PUSH foundation to arrange a boycott of Revlon, organize its symbolic funeral, and publicly criticize the company's presence in apartheid South Africa. Other initiatives, like the American Health and Beauty Aids Institute (AHBAI) Proud Lady Symbol on Black-owned products, tried to help Black customers more easily identify Black-owned companies and advance the goal of an economically self-sufficient Black community. Despite many efforts to re-politicize racial ownership, the numbers of Black-owned beauty businesses continued to dwindle through the 2000s.

Systemic gendered racism—evidenced by and perpetuated through racist and sexist representations of Black people, discriminatory financial institutions, and a dearth of resources catering to styling curly and coily hair textures—channeled Blacks into the less profitable salon servicing market. At the same time, these forces favorably positioning whites as manufacturers and Asians as suppliers in the more-lucrative manufacturing, retail, and distribution sectors of the Black beauty industry.[115] The shift to straight hairstyles facilitated Asian entrepreneurship in the Black beauty supply market as Black women's demands for weaves made with Indian, Chinese, and South Korean human hair rose. South Korean manufacturers gained a near monopoly on processing

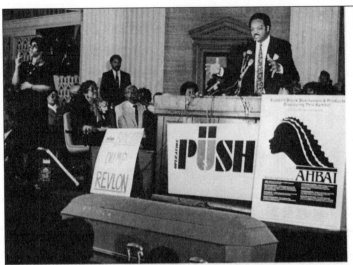

Rev. Jesse Jackson has called for a boycott of all Revlon products because of the company's racist statements about Blacks.

BUSINESS

PUSH Calls For Boycott Of Revlon, Holds 'Mock' Funeral

"Here lies Revlon dead because of greed," said the Rev. Jesse Jackson, "couldn't stand to watch Black businesses succeed."

Rev. Jackson's remarks were made at a mock funeral held at the Operation PUSH headquarters on Chicago's South Side to kick off a national boycott of all Revlon products and to symbolically dramatize the death of the Revlon cosmetics company.

14

At the front of the PUSH auditorium was a casket filled with Revlon products and draped with a floral arrangement which read:

Rev. Barrow, examines casket filled with Revlon products at mock funeral.

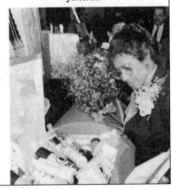

FIGURE 1.3. Reverend Jesse Jackson and Operation PUSH stage boycott against Revlon. Johnson Publishing Company Archive. Courtesy of Ebony Media LLC, the J. Paul Getty Trust, the Smithsonian National Museum of African American History and Culture, the Ford Foundation, the John D. and Catherine T. MacArthur Foundation, the Andrew W. Mellon Foundation, and the Smithsonian Institution.

human hair due to Korean government loans to the wig industry.[116] In the United States, Korean immigrants formed middleman businesses, using connections to human hair suppliers overseas to stock their beauty supply stores.[117] In the United States, Koreans came to enjoy 60% of the manufacturing, distribution, and retail market share of the Black beauty supply industry by the 2000s.[118] In places like the Netherlands, France, and Spain, Indian and Pakistani entrepreneurs established similar shops. To secure funding and circumvent bank loan processes that systematically excluded non-whites, immigrant social networks formed their own credit associations.[119]

Relationships between Blacks and Asians in the beauty supply industry demonstrate how white supremacy expresses itself through market dynamics, even in interactions between two non-white groups. George Lipsitz notes that conflict and cooperation "among racialized minorities [stems] from the recognition of the rewards of whiteness and the concomitant penalties imposed upon 'nonwhite' populations."[120] Korean American-owned beauty supply stores provide for and depend on Black consumers by stocking wide selections of hard-to-find products that Black American women want. In addition, some Black entrepreneurs collaborate with Asian manufacturers to create products for Black women. On the other hand, Korean immigrant success in the Black beauty market is often used to advance "model minority" myths that point to the economic mobility of some Asian Americans as proof of Black cultural deficiency, while deflecting attention away from distinct political and social realities—in this case, differential global trade networks and proximity to hegemonic feminine ideals for long, straight hair. Racial triangulation theory asserts that twin processes of relative valorization of Asian work ethic and Asian civic ostracism serve to maintain social and political white supremacy over people of both African and Asian descent in the United States.[121]

Triangulating Blacks and Asians as mutually inferior to whites but different from one another puts them in competition for resources. My interviewee Krystal worked for a Korean-owned beauty supply store in high school and recalled a conversation with a Black woman entrepreneur who was in competition with her employer: "She would explain to me how hard it was because certain companies won't sell to her when they realized she was African American. She was just like, there are laws in place and groups in place to prevent non-Korean store owners from getting products." A presenter at the 2015 Bronner Bros. International Hair Show made a similar accusation in a session about how to start a business importing human hair from China and India. The session was attended entirely by women of African descent, and the lead workshop facilitator was a middle-aged African American man who said that he had worked in the beauty industry for twenty years. He asserted, "Koreans come for one purpose. To sell hair to [Black people] from China. Chinese people get $17 million a month from the Koreans and are obligated to sell to the Koreans and not to Blacks. We [Black people] can't compete with $17 million." The presenter also warned the group about buying hair from Alibaba, a Chinese multinational e-commerce website worth billions of dollars, casting suspicion on Asian hair suppliers and feeding into xenophobic yellow peril metaphors that East Asians will conquer the West—triangulating Blacks and Asians by pitting Black American nativism against Asian perpetual foreignness. He then advised the group to try importing Indian hair instead, because he saw the market as less regulated and therefore more open to Black entrepreneurship. Black manufacturers, distributors, and retailers have collectively responded to real and perceived racial discrimination by Asian business owners through organizations like the Black Owned Beauty Supply Association (BOBSA), which aims to "connect the Black dots" within the beauty industry.

All in all, the shift in power over the Black beauty product manufacturing and retail industries away from Black entrepreneurs served to retrench the hegemony of Eurocentric feminine beauty ideals. As Ashley Mears well articulates in her study on determining factors of beauty in the fashion industry, "the relations of cultural production," taking into consideration modern markets, labor organization, decision-making

processes, and race and gender hierarchies, "determine the possibilities of cultural consumption."[122] Elizabeth Johnson's research shows
just that. Reading hair as text, she catalogued hairstyles shown in advertisements for *Ebony* and *Essence* magazines from 1985 to 2010 and
discovered that models' hairstyles in advertisements reflected the racial
ownership of the manufacturer.[123] Models for white-owned companies
tended be styled with straight hair, while Black-owned companies were
more likely to show models with natural hairstyles. Johnson argues that
white-owned manufacturers' cultural assumptions about beauty in the
ethnic haircare market idealize white femininity and decrease Black
women's options for alternative presentations of self. And so, as the new
millennium approached, Black women's hairstyling trends had almost
entirely shifted from Afros and cornrows to straight, long looks. The wet
and silky Jheri curl, chemical relaxers, and weaves were most popular
among Black women at the turn of the century.[124]

As the 2000s gave way to the 2010s, everything had changed, and yet
much was the same. Black women's economic insecurity and upward
mobility often continued to hinge upon their ability to embody cultural
assimilation and respectability. Heterosexual desirability continued to
be structured vis-à-vis Eurocentric norms. And yet, beauty remained
a space where Black women innovated to reflect who, where, and what
they wanted to be. The next chapter examines the continuing significance of race and hair in the twenty-first century, and how a burgeoning
natural hair culture online provided a new avenue for escape, rediscovery, and resistance.

2

Liberating Transitions

Cutting through Misogynoir

A recent graduate from a Historically Black College (HBCU) just entering the new, unfamiliar world of the corporate workforce, Keisha felt
at a confusing crossroads. She had just spent four years as a sociology
major critiquing how race, class, and gender bias impacted her K–12
education, reading feminist Marxism, and debating the merits of Booker
T. Washington and W. E. B. Du Bois's arguments about the best ways to
uplift the Black race. Alongside her intellectual transition into a Black
feminist political consciousness, Keisha was just on the other side of a
physical transition. She was one of a trickle of students on her campus
who had unveiled their natural zig-zagging curls, which had hibernated
for a year or so under weaves and braids, hair growth going unnoticed
under the plaits. Keisha's new look was not only well received, it was also
met with awe ("I wish I had the guts to do that!") and curiosity ("What
products are you using?") from her peers. These questions made her feel
beautiful and brave. While it turned out that many of her friends were,
in the quiet of their own dorm rooms, also feverishly scrolling through
YouTube videos by Black girls across the country who had somehow
experimented their way to shiny, healthy, kinky manes, Keisha was one
of the first who saw natural hair as possible for her, personally.

But college wasn't forever. Two years later, she was embarking on a career in corporate marketing. She quickly discovered that the norms gov-
erning the world outside her HBCU were much different, much more
confusing, than she expected. Having grown up in a predominately
Black neighborhood and gone to a predominantly Black college, this
was the first time she was going to be a minority in her environment,

and sometimes an "only." Should she—could she—be natural now? All the professional development seminars she'd attended in undergrad had warned her about needing to be twice as good, to speak Standard English, and the importance of owning a nice black, grey, or blue skirt suit. What about hair? She worried that her new kinky look would jeopardize her career mobility in her predominantly white company:

> I kind of conformed to the way Tiffany, the other Black lady who seems to be doing well at work on my team, was. Her hair is usually straight and it's very standardized. You know, American standardized hair—straight. She's natural as well, but she wears straight styles. Nice sleek buns, and so I thought for this current setting maybe my natural poofs and my natural hairstyles that I usually wear may not be as well received as they were at my HBCU because this is no longer an HBCU. This is a professional workplace and so I do find the weave . . . I mean I do have professional natural styles, but I've noticed that people have been more responsive to the responsible, to the weave or to the straight hair.

Keisha's concern reflects the reality that rejecting Eurocentric beauty standards continues to pose severe economic and social risks for Black people, particularly women, who are more likely than men to be measured by their appearance. In today's post-Civil Rights era, those with privilege frequently assert that people of all racial backgrounds now have equal access to opportunities, and thus, policies that consider race, even affirmatively, are inherently discriminatory. But race mobilizes vast cultural resources, symbols, and meanings that persist even after societies recognize their histories of slavery, imperialism, and exploitation. Ideological and material holdovers from centuries of explicit racial marginalization continue to privilege whites despite (and sometimes because of) non-racial policies. Ideas that straight hair is "standard," "responsible," and "professional" continue to undermine Black people like Keisha, even though none of these terms explicitly mention whiteness, Blackness, or race at all. Psychologist Leslie Carr calls this phenomenon "colorblind racism,"[1] and sociologist Eduardo Bonilla-Silva finds that in this context, whites increasingly employ alternative frames and stories that avoid explicitly invoking race while still making decisions that have racial and racist implications.[2] As Keisha's story highlights, aesthetics do not escape colorblind racism. Black people's exclusion from dominant perceptions of professionalism and beauty continues to politicize Black bodies well into this millennium. But, as this chapter will also discuss, digital technologies beget new strategies and frameworks for resistance. By the end of the 2010s, natural hair culture and its politics of authenticity had become a powerful new outlet for many Black women to try on new ways of being and seeing themselves over and against a multitude of pressures.

New Millennium, Same Misogynoir

Into the twenty-first century, discourses about and representations of Black hair in the media continue to reinforce many of the racist and sexist tropes of centuries past. For example, when radio talk show host Don Imus famously described the Rutgers University women's basketball team as "nappy-headed hos" in 2007, his remark dismissed the team's accomplishments as college students and award-winning athletes by using kinky hair to evoke racist stereotypes that Black women are hypersexual and unrespectable.[3] Similarly, at the 2015 Academy Awards, E! TV's Fashion Police cohost Giuliana Rancic commented that multiracial entertainer Zendaya's faux locs smelled like patchouli oil and weed, drawing race and class boundaries around the formal event that excluded Zendaya as inferior and potentially criminal because of her hair. In 2017, conservative pundit Bill O'Reilly rejected and minimized a critical speech African American congresswoman Maxine Waters delivered about then-President Donald Trump, stating, "I didn't hear a word she said, I was looking at the James Brown wig." O'Reilly's comments about Waters's hair relied upon racist and sexist stereotypes that Black women are too powerful and should be ignored if they cannot be silenced. Public figures like Imus, Rancic, and O'Reilly regularly reduce Black women's societal contributions through racist and sexist comments about their hair. By doing so on the public stage, the media and representatives of the state discipline and restrict Black women's presentations-of-self, maintain white middle-class feminine beauty standards, and reinforce white supremacy.

In addition, despite decades of critiques against workplace grooming policies banning popular Black hairstyles like cornrows, braids, and Afros, many colorblind but discriminatory rules continue to be newly instituted and upheld by the law. For example, in the spring of 2014, the United States Army updated its grooming policy to prohibit locs, twists, and large cornrows—all popular styles for managing Black hair during physical exercise. That the military policy described these styles as "unkempt" ignores the fact that cultural meanings of hair are racially constitutive and that professionalism and normative notions of attractiveness are racialized.[4] The military regulations were abandoned in February 2017 after widespread criticism by anti-racist advocates and Black women in the military, who made up 31% of all women enlisted in the Army during that time. However, similar policies are regularly upheld in state and federal courts. In September 2016, a US federal appeals court decision upheld an employers' right to ban loc'ed hair, arguing that the style is cultural and not racial in a biological sense, and thus not subject to protection by the Civil Rights Act of 1964. US Circuit Judge Alberto Jordan argued that, while hair texture is racialized and immutable, hairstyle is a "mutable characteristic of race."[5] Given that all hair textures are malleable, the court decision sent the message that non-white racialized phenotypes should be minimized. And in 2024, after the CROWN Act was passed to prevent hairstyle discrimination in schools and workplaces, a Texas judge ruled in favor of an independent school that punished a Black student for wearing his hair in locs due to their length. In this case, the gendered expectation that masculinity and long hair are mutually exclusive conveniently ignore a widely recognizable and culturally significant hairstyle among people of all genders across the

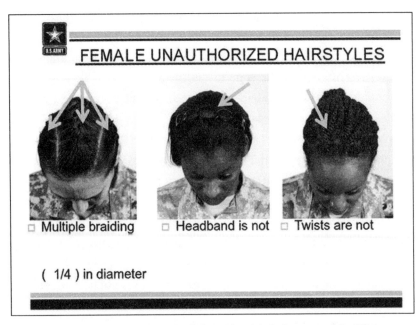

FIGURE 2.1. US Army Grooming Guidelines Visual Aid. Courtesy of the US Army.

African diaspora.[6] Employers' and administrators' attempts to control Black bodies at work produces "a particular effect—Black [people] remain visible yet silenced; their bodies become written by other texts," and they too often remain powerless to speak for themselves.[7]

Likewise, the United States Transportation Security Administration (TSA) regularly and disproportionately conducts pat downs of Black female travelers in particular, including searches of their natural hair. Pat downs of Black women's hair actually preceded enhanced security measures after the September 11, 2001 terrorist attacks. Per a 2000 US Government Accountability Office press release, Black women who are US citizens "were 9 times more likely than White women who were US citizens to be x-rayed after being frisked or patted town."[8] Sociologist Simone Browne theorizes the experience of state-sanctioned discrimination against Black and Brown people in airports as racial baggage, "where certain acts and certain looks at the airport weigh down some travelers, while others travel lightly."[9] Black women's bodies, especially those with natural hair, "come to represent, and also resist, security theater at the airport."[10] The presumed criminality of Black women in transit—their racial baggage—reflects punitive US War-on-Terror policies against non-whites, widespread Islamophobia, and white nativist xenophobia across the West in the early twenty-first century. It also reflects a long-standing fear and treatment of Black activist symbolism by government agencies and media outlets as defiant, un-American, and unpatriotic— from the 1970s Black Power era through to the ongoing Movement for Black Lives. This fear is a reaction to and backlash against a Black Power movement ideology, which politicized natural hair as symbolic of dia-sporic Black people's identification with an imagined African homeland, and relies on binary oppositional logic that had for centuries depicted the "cultured" West as superior to and inherently distinct from the "nat-urally" primitive "rest." The result? When Black women go natural, they become seen as incompatible with the (white) image of a naturalized American citizen. Or, in other words, agents of the state assume that a Black woman with natural hair must be a naturalized citizen from *else-where*, within a body politic to which they more "naturally" belong. This backlash increases Black women's racial baggage, while hair straighten-ing enables them to better navigate systemic gendered racism for easier spatial mobility.[11]

TSA searches are indiscriminate of class status and celebrity. In 2012, entertainer Solange Knowles tweeted about her experience of "Discrim-FRO-nation" at the airport, alongside a link to an article about TSA's public inspection of a woman named Isis Brantley's Afro, apparently for explosive material. I regularly have my natural hair searched by TSA agents and have been asked to remove a headscarf I wear to maintain my hairstyle. Usually, this entails a woman agent squeezing my hair into my head, or her running fingers from my forehead through my scalp. In March 2015, after the second of two similar complaints by Black women represented by the American Civil Liberties Union (ACLU), TSA agreed to begin training employees on the discriminatory impact of hair searches on Black women. ACLU Staff Attorney Novella Coleman explained in the press release announcing the agreement that "the humiliating experience of countless Black women who are routinely targeted for hair pat-downs because their hair is 'different' is not only wrong, but also a great misuse of time and resources."[12] However, explaining discriminatory impact to TSA agents does nothing to prevent or discourage discriminatory practices. This practice continues to be sheltered by laws that allow exceptions to unreasonable searches and discriminatory law enforcement based on race.

Even when Black women's bodies are not explicitly regulated, they remain pressured through conversations with friends, family, and co-workers to conform to a politics of respectability to find or keep jobs. For instance, at a 2017 panel discussion I attended about curls in the workplace, held at a coworking space in downtown Los Angeles, a featured panelist with natural hair explained to the audience how racialized professional norms affected her job hunt: "I was in the middle of a job search and I got a call for a job interview. I was at my friend's house and she gave me a straight bob wig to wear. This is sad that we have to do this. I don't know how it's going to be received or if it's going to be professional. I mean, by whose standard is it professional?" Her rhetorical question was met with grunts and nods of understanding from the audience. Friends and mothers of Black women often pass along their strategies for survival, socializing one another into a collective double consciousness to anticipate how Black hair is or might be seen by others. Zaire and Shauna, 23- and 24-year-olds living in Los Angeles, both described conversations with their mothers about how to wear their hair during job interviews. Zaire recalled, "My mom has made comments on 'oh you haven't found a job yet because you haven't combed your hair . . . She thinks that I shouldn't wear it out in an Afro. She thinks it will save my chances in the workplace." Shauna explained her mother's similar view of hair straightening as a proven strategy for upward mobility and economic advancement:

> For [my mom], growing up, hair was definitely straight because she wanted to move into a better life and going corporate and all that. For her, [it was] a no-brainer that her hair would have to be straight. When I started not to wear my hair that way it kind of threw her off because she didn't think it would be socially acceptable. She thought about how people think you are crazy and wild. She thought these things because that was something ingrained in her for her to get where she wanted to be.

Shauna's mother's reaction to her natural hair referenced white supremacist views that coily hair is a sign of Black women's inherent wildness; she saw straight hair as one way to protect her daughter's right to employment, dignity, and civil life.

Caribbean women interviewees also described how colorism and texturism shape their lives. For example, Gina, a 47-year-old Afro-Surinamese and Guyanese woman in Amsterdam, noted the Caribbean idea of encouraging children to "*opo yu kloro*," or "open up your color." In other words, *opo yu kloro* means to pursue romantic relationships with lighter-skinned partners to increase one's chance of having children with closer-to-white features. Gina told me:

> My grandmother, who was of mixed race from British Guyana, and one of my aunts disliked my mother because of her darker skin color. My grandmother even fainted when she first saw my mother's picture. How could her favorite son move to Europe and choose a woman whose skin is darker than his? They were actually relieved when my parents divorced and my father is now married to a woman with a light skin color and straight hair. My grandmother's sister was married to a Chinese man so her children have Asian features (one of her granddaughters was at my birthday with her family). When one of her daughters moved to the USA

and my grandmother's sister found out she was dating an African American she took a flight to take her daughter back home. Sad isn't it?

While Gina proudly wears her locs around family, her half-sister has been effectively disowned by the other side of her family for wearing her hair out in an Afro. Gina's personal family history of racial mixing and international migration across the Black Atlantic highlights the ongoing, transcultural, and transgenerational conversations that Africana communities have around race and beauty politics.

Jane, a 42-year-old media executive from Los Angeles, took cues from more senior Black women in her field when deciding how to wear her hair at work. In our interview, Jane recalled a subtle conversation with her boss about how she should wear her hair for an upcoming presentation to executives. She told me, "I remember one day I was wearing [my hair] natural and big and my boss at the time was Black, she's mixed, she's from New York and I was like 'should I not do this tomorrow?' She would have never said no but she was like 'ehh I think I'm going to press mine' and I was like alright." Jane learned and accepted that straight hairstyles are key to upward mobility in the workplace. As her reflections demonstrate, racist stereotypes that Black hair is wild and unprofessional and respectability politics from the mid-twentieth century continue to inform Black women's hair politics. Such insecurities are especially acute for Black women in a neoliberal era of deregulation, as individuals are increasingly held privately responsible for making themselves marketable and, in turn, socially successful, despite stratifying social systems of capitalism, racism, and patriarchy, as well as increasing labor precarity. Psychologists Adrienne Evans and Sarah Riley explain that "the management of risk within the discourses of neoliberal femininity presents women as always culpable for their own individualized failure, often in highly racialized and classed ways."[13]

Many women's concerns that their natural hairstyles will hinder their careers are reinforced by their interactions at work. When Michelle, a 49-year-old from Los Angeles stopped straightening her hair for health reasons, she was ostracized by her coworkers. She told me, "When I first started wearing [my hair in] puffs and trying to come up with my own flavor I would walk in a room at work and I could see all eyes on me and it wasn't like, 'aww that's great!' it was like '*what* is she *doing*?' and I had to like, push through all of that."

Paula, a 26-year-old living in Los Angeles, confronted the controlling image of the mammy when she wore her hair in a head wrap to work. Her experience demonstrates that centuries-old racist representations of Black womanhood continue to shape interactions in the twenty-first century:

> One time I wore a wrap for the first time and when I did wear a turban, I remember the security guy at the front desk . . . the first thing he said was do you have any syrup? I'm like huh? It's early morning and I'm confused. I'm not as sharp as I am around two pm. I'm like, huh? And he's like Aunt Jemima! I was like literally . . . I wanted to go off. I just said no and walked to my desk. Come on! That was one thing that really, really annoyed me.

This interaction was a microaggression, a term that refers to the everyday subtle statements, behaviors, and environments—whether intentional or not—that communicate derogatory or hostile beliefs based on the identity of a target group.[14] While microaggressions may seem minor or trivial, they maintain the white supremacist and patriarchal status quo by silencing, excluding, and marginalizing their target.

Women I interviewed in South Africa described similar workplace dynamics. Brie, 35-year-old university administrator from Cape Town, told me that her coworkers' comments about her hair silenced her from participating in meetings despite her desire to contribute:

> I was in [Johannesburg] two weeks ago for a conference and there are so many things I could have spoken about, but I also keep quiet about insecurity and not feeling like I was fully part of the team. But it was also a case that they dismissed what I have to say and, "oh you didn't go with

your hair like that to the meeting" or whatever. It feeds into it. Like, it trips you up! It is hard being a woman of color at the moment for me.

In post-apartheid South Africa, where corporate workplaces are slowly diversifying, macro-level shifts are felt through interpersonal interactions which discipline women's presentations-of-self. Marley, a 26-year-old teacher in Cape Town, illustrated this in our interview:

> Where I am working now it is a private school, very strict. I have to be precise with what I want to do. The other night we went to a very fancy restaurant, and they come around and then there were African dancers that come while you are eating, and you taste traditional dishes and it is made very well. At the end of the night, they throw dust on the people and they are like, "experience the gold of Africa." My coworker told me, maybe the dust will be magical and your hair will be straight tomorrow. I didn't say much because I'm new to the company and I didn't want them to hate me but I felt very insulted by that. Why do you want my hair straight? Why do you think it should be straight? It could be a race thing because she was white and I am Coloured. The company that I work for is majority white people and they feel like the Coloured people are taking over and I'm in a management position. I still rocked it at work like girl please I'm not going to change for you. Who are you? No! But I thought about wearing braids for a month and I wondered whether I shouldn't now. I don't want to think about what I must do next, I just want to be. Why can't I be? Let me just be.

The comment by Marley's coworker is a classic example of colorblind racism. Because Marley's coworker never explicitly mentioned race, Marley had to guess her coworker's intention. So, Marley left the inter-action without a clear sense of whether she has the right to demand an apology or file a grievance against her coworker even though she felt deeply insulted and disrespected. Instead, Marley unfairly took on an insecurity about her hair and a fear of being disliked—of being seen as angry and hostile. The interaction taught her to self-police her style at work moving forward. The interaction was even more powerful given where it took place—the colleague was happy to be entertained with African culture at a restaurant, but implied that Marley's hair was unwelcome in the predominantly white professional setting they shared. These sorts of interactions produce a particular effect, telling women of color where they should be and where they do not belong. In places with histories of European settler colonialism and displacement like South Africa, such comments are interpersonal forms of colonialism where white elites take space, dignity, and the right to expression away from people of color, thus reinforcing white supremacy.

Outside of the office, race and gender also intersect with sexuality to shape how beauty politics work in the dating market. As beauty scholar Kristin Denise Rowe points out, Black queer women reimagine and embody beauty in ways that decenter a heteronormative male gaze but exist within a larger context of cisnormativity.[15] The ability to "pass" as cis can sometimes rely on an acquiescence to feminine norms idealizing long hair. So, while beauty norms have tended to be more flexible in queer communities, they are also often formed vis-à-vis persistent heteronormativity and homophobia. Sociologist Mignon Moore's research on gender display in Black lesbian communities found that "femme aggressive" and "transgressive" lesbians, or Black lesbians who gender-blend by rocking more masculine presentations, are more likely to wear buzz cuts, locs, twists, and other natural hairstyles.[16] In a conversation analyzing their personal experiences with Black lesbian beauty, writers Jennifer Lyle, Jeanell Jones, and Gail Drakes contemplated how the rise of 1990s Afrocentrism challenged the association of natural hair with a Black lesbian identity. Jones wondered:

> Right now, in Black culture, we're going through a whole change of trying to look more Afrocentric—an interesting change is emerging. What we identify as a Black lesbian is often a person who wears her hair natural,

uses no makeup, and wears "dreads." I wonder how those images are now regarded; if it's gonna make straight Black folk think they might be misidentified as queer.[17]

Then and now, natural hair is widely considered outside the realm of heterosexual desirability. (In fact, several of the heterosexual women I interviewed wondered whether short hair or natural hair might erode their desirability to male romantic prospects and current romantic partners.) But many lesbian and queer women choose masculine haircuts to protect themselves from being desired and pursued by heterosexual men.[18] And, even as butch Black queer women find connection and expression through those communal norms, discrimination, prejudice, and the threat of violent homophobia police binary gender self-presentations and discourage some women from outwardly signaling a lesbian identity through hair and dress.[19] Narrow understandings of feminine beauty put extra pressure on Black trans women to "do womanhood" appropriately to avoid discrimination. As writer Ivana Fischer wrote in a 2020 article reflecting on her relationship with her natural hair for the *Huffington Post*:

> For Black trans women like me, this can be an extremely difficult conundrum to navigate. We are bombarded with prejudice based on preconceived notions about our gender identities and how we *should* present. For us to go without rocking a few extra inches in—at the very least, a cheap Shake-n-Go—would constitute an invitation for every aspect of our biologies to be called into question. From our body types, to our muscle densities, to the amount of base in our voices, Black trans women are too often picked apart and ridiculed. If you think Black cisgender women are held to the most unforgiving societal standards of natural beauty, think again.[20]

As feminist philosopher Judith Butler's incisive portrait of violence against intersex and trans communities and sociologist Patricia Hill

Collins's analysis of Sakia Gunn's murder both demonstrate, bodies that transgress social norms are often excluded, marginalized, put at risk, and are thus inherently political.[21] Given the overt and implicit ways Black women are systematically held accountable to a hegemonic heterofemininity that devalues Blackness, it is evident that hair and beauty remain social justice concerns.

If stigmas against and surveillance of Black bodies in the twenty-first century remain consistent with conditions of the past, the ability for Black communities to respond has broadened, thanks to the advent of social media and the rise of vocal natural hair and other political and identity-based communities on- and offline. A confluence of shifts in the political economy, technology, and popular culture in the late 2000s allowed natural hair to become a full-blown lifestyle movement among women of African descent. In 2008, Chris Rock's documentary *Good Hair* revived a conversation about the politics of Black hair on an international level. The film explored the physical, emotional, and financial toll that straightening hair to appeal to white beauty ideals takes on Black women's lives. While *Good Hair* harshly critiqued wearing weaves and using chemical relaxers, it left viewers unsettled, without clear pathways for change. The rise of visually-oriented, web 2.0 social media platforms filled the gap that *Good Hair* left behind. YouTube (released 2005), Tumblr (2009), and Instagram (2010), enabled previously isolated Black women to form virtual communities and exchange information about styling natural hair, concocting products at home, and fostering self-acceptance. Digital conversations about wellness, beauty, and Black empowerment spilled offline and into kitchens, bathrooms, beauty shops, and convention centers around the world, transforming the way Black women saw, cared for, and felt about themselves. As blogging and vlogging surged, Black women created and discovered new images of natural hair. Proto-influencers like Nikki Walton of CurlyNikki.com, Patrice Yursick of Afrobella.com, and Leila Noelliste of BlackGirlLongHair.com posted pictures of their natural hair journeys to their websites and YouTube channels, shared recipes for homemade hair potions made with avocado and honey, and modeled a confidence that felt new, fresh, and authentic. Onlookers got curious about their own natural hair textures and rethought their regimens. Could they be natural, too?

Transitioning: A New Politics of Authenticity

Up until the 2010s, most Black women received their first chemical relaxers as children and had not seen or cared for their natural hair texture for years or even decades.[22] So natural hair spaces, at least at the beginning, focused heavily on the practice of purging permanently straightened hair to reveal its natural hair texture—a process that became known as *transitioning*. Women usually transition to natural hair in one of two ways. The first way is by growing out chemically relaxed or heat-damaged hair over an extended period, and gradually cutting off the straight ends to retain a desired hair length. The point where virgin hair meets processed hair is called the *line of demarcation*. The process of transitioning is complete when one's hair has been trimmed to this point. Hair growth is a slow process; it can take several months for women with tightly coiled hair to discover their natural texture. Women might braid, weave, twist, or heat-style their hair during this time to camouflage the difference in texture between their curly new hair growth and their straighter processed ends. For example, Michelle (49, Los Angeles) wore straight weaves during her transition while her natural hair grew underneath. Later, she switched to box braids to avoid heat damage caused by thermally pressing her edges to match the texture of the weave. Every couple of months, she'd take down her weave, cut off an inch or two of her relaxed hair, and then have her stylist install a new weave. After six months, Michelle was ready to debut her new, natural hairdo.

Another way women transition to natural hair is by getting a *big chop*, a term from natural hair culture that refers to the practice of shaving off all of one's hair at once for an immediate, fresh start. In the opening poem to this study, "Wild Crown," I. S. Jones conjures this practice in the first line, "chop me from the neck up," and later in the poem, she refers to her newly-barren scalp. While a general search for "transitioning natural hair" shows about 580 thousand results on YouTube, a search for "big chop" garners over 4.6 million hits, highlighting the importance of this practice to natural hair culture, as well as the spectacle it has become. Big chopping is dramatic in its abruptness, and seen as brave for going against cultural norms. Rose Weitz calls baldness "the ultimate 'in your face' hair statement" for women in Western heteronormative and patriarchal societies because it eschews feminine beauty norms of long hair and blurs cultural signifiers of masculinity and femininity. She finds that generally, rebellious, politically radical, or artistic women choose the style, as do women who want to signal a lesbian identity.[23] An intersectional analysis mindful of how racism and heteronormativity shape women's lives must also note the cultural impact of head-shaving as a form of punishment and shame during slavery, homophobic associations between short hair and feminine desirability, and the centrality of hair style, texture, and length to Black women's cultural, social and personal identities.[24] Within this context, transitioning to natural hair by big chopping can be shocking for both the person who does it and those around them. Maria, a panelist at an intimate natural hair forum discussion about the experience of transitioning to natural hair, told the group about severe pushback from her family when she big chopped because she rejected conventional heterofeminine beauty and respectability ideals. She recalled:

> My family looked at me different. They thought I was this wild child, you know, being from the South where you can't talk back to your parents. My uncle told me that this style was for men. That's dyke. Dyke women wear that! And it kind of stabbed me in my chest. I was getting all these energies from my family and now all the sudden I'm different. So, I wore this shirt to be a superwoman that said "I heart my hair."

Patriarchal homophobia makes "going natural" a risky choice, potentially putting women in danger of emotional and physical harm. But Maria's testimony also reveals that the practice of big chopping can be liberating and self-affirming. Against much hurt and disappointment from her family, Maria asserted the "superwoman" within herself.

Regardless of the method of becoming natural, most women I interviewed describe transitioning to natural hair as both an external and internal process of self-discovery. As Candis F. Tate explains, "the process of transitioning is important to evaluate because it is the first step in many Black women's natural hair journey. Transitioning begins an entirely new process of handling and caring for Black hair, and more importantly, it is a critical stage where Black women beg[i]n fostering a new relationship with hair."[25] For these reasons, Black women often describe the experience of letting their hair grow out naturally as revelatory. 62-year-old Corliss in Charlotte, NC was transitioning when we spoke. She wore her hair in a straight pressed style when she was a child, then relaxed it from seventh grade until three months prior to our interview. She exclaimed, "The new phase I'm in, I haven't seen my hair like this since I was a little girl. Or ever! I haven't seen my hair like this ever!"

This emphasis on transitioning—going from one way of looking, doing, and being seen to another way of looking, doing, and being seen—is a distinct element of contemporary natural hair politics, though curiously absent from discussions about the Afro in the 1960s and 1970s. Perhaps this distinction speaks to a difference between natural hair as symbol then, and natural hair as journey now. Activists and scholars often describe the Afro as part of the Black Power "uniform of rebellion," a signal that portrayed someone's Afrocentric political orientation to others. In contrast, women in the natural hair movement describe becoming natural as an intimate, personal journey to learn and be who they are from the outside in. Fannie (45, Los Angeles) explained:

I will say that in the '70s it was probably more of an "I'm Black and I'm proud," you know? It was like a revolution. It was like, I have to fight to take a stance for my rights. This time it's "I like me." I just love my hair this way and I don't care what anybody thinks.

Typical of new social movements like the peace and gay rights movements, the natural hair movement emphasizes individual autonomy and self-transformation compared with traditional social movements, like the labor and Civil Rights movements, which tend to operate through formal organizations that target state-level redistributive change.

For me, loving my natural hair came with confidence. I'm so out. This is who I am. This is me. I want to wear the bright purple lipstick and the earrings and look at me. This is who I am. This is me and I'm proud to be it. I remember not wanting attention but then I got confidence with myself. It was more so an acceptance thing. Fully becoming comfortable in my own skin to want to. (Paula, 27, Los Angeles)

It took a lot of perseverance—I still have a few straight bits here and there and I'm supposed to go for a trim later on—but I just feel more confident. It's weird. When I walk, I like the stares now. I used to hide away. Now I can't wait because I'm owning this and whoever doesn't like it it's their problem and for a long time I shielded away from it but up until last week my aunt was here and she was like, "Your hair, when are you going to do it? When are you going to do your hair? It's not attractive." I feel like this is my hair and whoever doesn't accept it, to hell with them. (Brie, 35, Cape Town)

As these illustrations of self-love and confidence emphasize, going natural is not just a physical experience. For many women, the emotional aspect of transitioning is just as significant, if not more. Becoming natural forces many women to notice their distance from and internalization of mainstream beauty ideals, which continue to underrepresent dark-skinned women and women with kinky hair. It took months for Krystal to view her natural hair texture as beautiful and worthy. Krystal had worn her hair chemically relaxed since elementary school and in long, wavy weaves once she could afford them. She recalled:

> It was hard! I remember it being very, very hard. I didn't know how it would turn out. I didn't know if my hair texture would be something I would like—my natural hair texture. I didn't know how to really manage my natural hair coming in with my relaxed hair. I didn't know a lot of stuff about my hair and I didn't want to deal with it.

When Krystal realized she could not change her hair texture without chemicals or heat, she learned to, in her words, "get with the program." Getting with the program catalyzed the beginning of a new way of thinking about her body and made her critical of what her beauty practices insinuated about her self-esteem:

> It's like, the more I think about it . . . I got into a relationship with my natural hair and the closer I got in the relationship with my natural hair the more deviated I was from my connection to the weave even though the connection was near and dear to my heart. The thought of putting someone else's hair in my head because oh, it's convenient? It's like, am I that desperate to have a look that I would wear the actual follicles off of someone else's hair? You have to use somebody else's *actual hair* to put in *your hair* because it's *convenient* or it *makes you feel better.*

Krystal's reflections make it clear that transitioning is not simply a physical embrace of one's natural hair texture; transitioning also inspires critical inquiry of societal beauty standards and one's own emotional state.

Moreover, Krystal personified her hairstyles, coming to see her weave as a being of its own that separated her from a healthy, authentic relationship with her inner self. When I asked her when she felt the most beautiful, Krystal replied:

I feel the most beautiful, like [pause] at any point at this point. I say that because since I know me wearing my Afro, I've grown into a relationship with my Afro and this is just me. I'm unapologetically me when I have my Afro. When I came out of my mother's womb, this is how my hair began to grow. This is how it is. This is me at my core being. I can appreciate and love myself as who I am, how I wake up in the morning and my hair is just goofy. I can love and appreciate my hair when it's straight because I know who I am and I appreciate who I am at my core now. It's a relationship that I didn't have when I first was natural but eventually I grew into it. I fell in love with my natural hair at some point, and it tells me to love me with a weave, me with a press-out, me with a twist-out, me on my bad hair days.

Interestingly, Krystal does not describe natural hair as a uniform of rebellion or an outward political symbol. Transitioning transcended her physical appearance and extended to her "core being." Likewise, Fannie (45) talks about the power of accepting one's natural hair texture this way:

Basically, natural is being comfortable in your own skin, in your own body, with your own hair, your own look, you know? It's just being comfortable with your texture of hair. So, you can rock a natural hairstyle and it not be your [own hair] . . . it cannot look like your texture and be altered and still be a natural hairstyle *look* but a lot of people find that their confidence is actually coming from them actually rocking their own hair. And then after you get the hang of your own hair you love that and you feel confident and secure in that then you can play. You can play with different things. Natural is basically you loving and liking your own-ness. Having your own hair. Just being in love with that. Your Blackness, your beauty, your curves, your hair, your skin. That to me is natural.

Transitioning, according to these women, is an inner journey from insecurity to confidence with the final destination being a level of self-confidence that persists through any form of creative hair play. This emphasis on self-love suggests that authenticity, rather than Afrocentrism, is a defining priority in contemporary natural hair culture.

Some women describe feeling immediately liberated from social norms dictating identity and appearance upon big chopping. Lauren (26, New York City) told me:

> The first day that I wore my hair after getting it cut, the first day that I actually went out of the house and everything I just felt so amazing. I was just so okay in my own skin. Nothing special really happened that day but that was one of the best days of my life. Is that weird? It was so long that I went without being okay in my own skin feeling like I should be different, a little thicker, all these little tweaks and when you are finally like you know what, I like me, that feels damn good.

She showed me the first photo she took of herself after her big chop, laying in her bed and smiling with her TWA—"teeny weeny Afro." She had posted the photo to her Instagram account a few months before our interview and grinned as she pulled it up on her iPhone to show me. These women's declarations of joy and self-love within and against a racist and sexist society are political in and of themselves. They are also crucial to Black women's potential for community-wide change. After all, "[Black women] cannot create effective movements for social change if individuals struggling for that change are not also self-actualized or working towards that end."[26]

Lindi (41, Cape Town) also told a transition story that focused on confidence and self-esteem. She decided to transition to natural hair because she saw her daughter's self-worth crumble due to ruthless teasing of her *bossiekop* (kinky) hair by her cousins with straighter hair. Lindi came to believe she was reinforcing her daughter's insecurities by relaxing her and her daughter's hair. She told me:

> When I started off my natural hair, or return to natural as I call it, it wasn't for any political reason. It was because of my daughter. I started relaxing

her hair at the age of five, which is bad. Now I can see that it was wrong but back then it was normal. Back when I was little it was normal. I was scared because in my community, in the Coloured community, this was unheard of . . . This is what they call *bossiekop*. This is the term that is used. Derogatory terms. I was at the point where I could no longer lie to myself and it needed to be done. We transitioned for a year. We did it together, and then we eventually cut it off. I cut my hair first and allowed her to make up her mind about it.

Hair was a gateway for Lindi to critique power relations within her community that marginalized those with curlier hair textures. Realizing how deeply texturism influenced her daughter's self-esteem, Lindi gave her daughter daily affirmations. She recalled, "I would boost her confidence . . . I would say things like 'gosh you are so stunning and so intelligent and I love your hair' . . . eventually she became this powerhouse of a child where she was fighting her own battles." Lindi's neighbors' and family members' disdainful comments about her hair texture brought her attention to aspects of Coloured culture that she wanted to change. She continued, "As far as the political thing, it came in a bit later because as you wear your hair natural, as you go you kind of realize what it all stands for. You realize that it is about your culture. That it's not a fashion statement . . . There's so much more to the point where sometimes I can be quite militant about it." As Lindi's experience reveals, an embodied transition can ultimately become politicizing. Being a woman of African descent is not necessarily a fixed identity standpoint, but a self-conscious location from which to see. As women's embodiments shift, so too do their standpoints, or their ways of looking at themselves and the world. Such shifts in standpoint are not necessarily inevitable or immediate, but as Lindi's reflection shows, they can produce new, critical, and political insights.

For Lola (26, Bahia), transitioning to natural hair entailed an understanding of herself as part of a Black collective political identity for the first time. The meaning of her transition to natural hair stems from the history of race and construction of Blackness in Brazil. She explained:

> Belonging to the Black race is built under negative stereotypes, so we are taught from an early age that our hair is bad, ugly, and that we must modify it to be socially valued in the labor market. In this way, a good part of Brazilian Black women, including me, straighten their hair early in childhood, but the traces of belonging cannot be changed, such as skin color. So, I spent fifteen years of my life smoothing my hair, did not know what the natural root was, and because of this that I did not recognize myself as a Black woman, but from the moment I became aware of the meaning of racism, and how he acted in my body, I decided to stop smoothing my hair. I began to recognize myself within an ethnic and political identity, to be a Black woman. From then on, I experienced a new identity, when I cut my hair straight and saw the natural grow, I saw myself Black for the first time, and unlike what I was taught, I found myself beautiful.[27]

Brazil projects itself as a "racial democracy," a country where citizens do not see themselves or each other through the lens of race.[28] In this context, Lola's description of coming to a Black identity through the process of transitioning to natural hair is quite striking. For her, transitioning was a decolonial act, a way of undoing her embodied internalization of racism that considers Black phenotypical identifiers ugly and bad. Not only did her feelings about her natural appearance change, but she also came to see herself as part of a collective political and racial identity. Lola asked about my own experience with natural hair, and I mentioned to her the difficulty of navigating work and relationships. This inspired her to clarify a difference between the effect of natural hair in Brazil and in the United States:

> The women here in Brazil leave their hair natural, for reasons very similar to those that you point out in the reality of the United States, but I believe that the identity factor is what prevails, or political declaration,

that refers to the perception of belonging to a common origin, to an ethnic group, where, from the moment they realize that they are exposed to a particular type of oppression, they have been empowered to get out of this situation.

Lola's insights are mirrored by Elizabeth Hordge-Freeman's study on racial features, socialization, and affective experiences in Brazilian families. Hordge-Freeman finds that hair texture is more decisive for racial identification than skin color or body shape in Brazil, and that transitioning to natural hair functions as a rite of passage for those who choose to "*assumir-se*" (assume their Blackness).[29]

Black Beauty Politics 2.0

Virtual natural hair communities are often women's first layer of practical and emotional support during the process of transition and amid their public debuts with natural hair. Many women shared with me how Facebook groups, Instagram accounts, YouTube influencers, and Pinterest boards helped them to find pride in their hair, learn new styling practices, and create community with like-minded Black women in their local communities and well beyond. Brie, 35, explained the impact of a Cape Town-based Facebook group for women with natural hair, in which hundreds of new messages are posted daily: "Being part of that group that I'm in on Facebook where [natural hair] is acceptable, you don't feel alone because of the transition. Transitioning was hard. It's painful actually because you're very tempted to go back." Marley, 26, participates in two local natural hair online forums, and also mentioned their usefulness:

> I get a lot of support from the natural ladies on Facebook. Confidence to look the way I want to and be free because there were so many times where I felt ugly and I can't walk out like this and I can't be seen like this and then these ladies just motivated me because they took raw pictures

in the bathroom and I saw that okay, I'm not that bad. It is nice to have people to share an experience with you.

Likewise, Lauren (26, New York) told me, "I follow @TheCutLife on Instagram and some natural pages that just have random pictures of people with natural hair. Just seeing oh, I can do that style, or to keep you motivated because being natural isn't always . . . when you see things that are working for other people it helps you to stay strong." Having tagged her own big chop photo with the hashtags #naturalhair, #Blackgirlmagic, and #bigchop, Lauren's selfie became searchable to the rest of the digital blogosphere, paying forward encouragement to other women of color who might likewise be searching for role models absent from their immediate physical communities. Online natural hair communities, hashtags, and accounts serve as grassroots archives that disseminate resistant Black aesthetics, and everyday women often unintentionally become contributors to this cache.

Much feminist scholarship on beauty argues that patriarchy and its capitalist mode of production rely on unachievable beauty ideals and exploit the gap between advertising images of women and women's actual bodies to sell products.[30] However, these kinds of feminist analyses sidestep women's agency as cultural producers and consumers. What happens when corporations compete with everyday people for control over image production? In the digital age, Black women have access to and are creating new platforms to publicly share their experiences of hair discrimination and what it feels like for others to casually treat their bodies as public property. For example, designer Momo Pixel's interactive computer game *Hair Nah* went viral in 2017.[31] In the game, the player first assembles a character from a range of brown skin tones and natural hairstyles. After choosing a destination, the player defends the character's natural hair using the arrow keys to swat a barrage of light-complexioned grabbing hands away. The game's outro reads, "The game is over, but this experience isn't. This is an issue that Black women face daily. So, note to those that do it: STOP THAT SHIT."

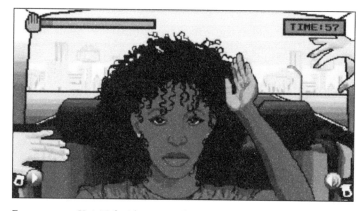

FIGURE 2.2. *Hair Nah* video game character swats strangers' hands from petting her natural hair. Courtesy of Momo Pixel.

Social media influencers demonstrate how to transition, choose products, style natural hair, and grow confidence in the wake of persistent social pressures. For instance, Nikki Walton of CurlyNikki.com, Patrice Yursik of Afrobella.com, and Whitney White of @Naptural85 on YouTube have huge international followings. Online natural hair communities are sizeable. The Facebook group South African Naturals boasts 121,000 members. The Brazilian Facebook group *Poder Crespo/Dicas E Transição* has attracted almost 13,000 members and is steadily growing after a successful street protest in Salvador, Bahia. The US-based website and forum NaturallyCurly.com has received over 611,000 Facebook likes. In November 2017, the site's founder reported reaching 16 million readers monthly. A simple search for "natural hair" on YouTube garners over 8.7 million results. Digital platforms like these have become archives of natural hair culture. These virtual communities disseminate natural hair practices, norms, and a set of terms that reimagine the old Black hair lexicon.[32] Tiffany M. Gill suggests that natural hair communities on social media may come to supplement—or even supplant—the role that beauty shops played in fostering Black women's activism in the twentieth century.[33] The natural hair movement is Black beauty politics 2.0, and Black women increasingly use digital media technology to facilitate discussion, sisterhood, and collective action. As one natural hair blogger on a panel at the 2015 Afrolicious Hair Affair natural hair expo in Los Angeles declared, "If it's on the media it doesn't validate us; it doesn't mean that's validation for how we should be. We are just as powerful as the women on *Vogue* or the women on *Scandal*."

The Perception Institute's 2017 "Good Hair" study suggests that online natural hair communities significantly influence how Black women see themselves. The study found that Black women who participate in online natural hair communities are more likely than Black or white women who do not to prefer or have positive attitudes toward Black women wearing textured hairstyles.[34] They suggest that natural hair blogs, vlogs, message boards, and forums transform Black women's views about hair texture: "engagement with the [natural hair] community, beyond just personal ideas about natural hair, may be a method of reducing implicit biases and warrants further study."[35] Elizabeth Johnson likewise finds that blogs aid some Black women in imagining solidarity with other women based on hair texture.[36] Tameka Ellington has also documented how African American women use social media networks to form support groups when they lack resources or advice elsewhere, sharing strategies for navigating schools, the workplace, and resistance from romantic partners.[37]

Conclusion

Misogynoir remains alive and well into the twenty-first century, but new tools and technologies have given way to new critiques by Black women—both in form and in function. In a web-2.0 world, Africana women are using YouTube, Pinterest, Facebook, Tumblr, Instagram, and independent websites to create and discover more authentic and affirming ways of being and presenting. Early natural hair influencers became grassroots role models who supplemented and supplanted mainstream representations of beauty that more powerful corporations produced and circulated. These influencers shared images and stories about how they transitioned away from chemical relaxers, how they came to find self-acceptance, and how they learned to care for their kinky and curly natural hair. Millions of Black women curiously scrolled on their smartphones, tablets, and laptops. The simple fact of their own curiosity became evidence that natural hair really could be desirable—if not to romantic partners or HR departments, then to Black women themselves. In the process, a new racial project—the natural hair movement—was born.

As Black women around the world transitioned and big chopped their ways to natural hair, they faced workplaces and dating markets that foregrounded Eurocentric beauty standards and the heterosexual male gaze. They also ran up against deep worries and insecurities that their natural bodies wouldn't be beautiful enough, strong enough, or smart enough to navigate the persistent gendered racism around them. Because of those challenges, the women I interviewed tended to describe their natural hair journeys as vehicles of self-love and self-care. This emphasis on self-acceptance represents an emerging Black feminist politics of authenticity and distinguishes the new natural hair movement from ways that Black women have used beauty to embody resistance in the past. While a politics of respectability saw natural hair as a barrier to cultural assimilation and a politics of Afrocentricity saw natural hair as a symbolic counter-embrace of imagined African values, a politics of authenticity sees natural hair as a vehicle for Black women to learn to love themselves as they are despite external pressures. This politics of authenticity is a distinguishing feature of contemporary natural hair and Black beauty politics.

3

Green Is the New Black

Naturalness as a Wellness Project

I sat sipping a cup of coffee at an outdoor café in the trendy hipster Maboneng neighborhood of Johannesburg, South Africa while I waited for my interview with Sheila, the 45-year-old owner of a line of hair- and skincare products marketed toward women with natural hair. Sheila was a petite, brown-skinned woman with a halo of tightly coiled curls that glistened in the sun. When she turned the corner, her glow seemed to reach me before the rest of her body did. As Sheila settled in her seat across from me at our sidewalk table, I waved over the waiter so she could place her order. She politely declined my invitation to purchase her a drink as a thank you for making the time to chat. She explained, "Caffeine is a drug. I've always been conscious about what I put in my body." She went on to describe her history of unsuccessful yo-yo dieting, the homemade detox brew of bentonite clay and kale she was exclusively drinking, and how her overall embrace of a plant-based approach to eating and cosmetics has changed her life. She boasted further that her daughter "is thinner than the thinnest girl, but she's very assertive so it doesn't really bother her because she says [the girls at school] want to look like [her]." As our interview progressed, Sheila expounded that she uses her hair and skincare company's sales pitch to extend the conscious veganism she practices with her family to the broader Black community. Her perspective was not uncommon among the women I met within natural hair spaces, and represents an emerging form of aesthetic labor and entrepreneurship among Black women today that brings green politics and Black politics together.

During the week that I interviewed Sheila in August 2016, the news cycle in South Africa alternated between protests at a nearby high school against policies that prohibited students from wearing natural hair and debates around a proposed 20% tax on sugar-sweetened drinks as a strategy to combat obesity, which affects 40% of women and 11% of men in South Africa.[1] While the media did not tie these two issues together, Sheila explicitly discussed natural hair as a healthcare practice. Though she had one of the more extreme alternative lifestyle regimens among my interviewees, her story of increased concern about diet, fitness, and exposure to harmful chemicals was common among women I interviewed in South Africa and elsewhere. This was part of, and maybe even a catalyst to, an intensifying overlap between beauty politics, wellness politics, and racial politics. Some women's worries about chemical toxicity preceded their transitions away from hair relaxers because health challenges like weight gain, diabetes, cancer, or high blood pressure necessitated alterations in their diet, exercise, and beauty regimens. As the natural hair movement progressed, many of these women's concerns were validated by new research tying relaxers to breast and uterine cancers, culminating in a set of class action lawsuits against cosmetics companies in the 2020s.[2] Other women described learning about a wide range of wellness practices—from breastfeeding to nutritional literacy—through their participation in natural hair communities.

An emphasis on health and wellness is a defining feature of contemporary Black women's beauty politics, and increasingly, of mainstream beauty politics in the twenty-first century. In contrast to twentieth-century Black beauty culturists who promoted hair straightening as a form of respectability politics and Black Power and Black Consciousness activists who wore Afros as an outward signifier of a commitment to an Afrocentric worldview, many women transitioning to natural hair in the twenty-first century say the catalyst for their choice is maintaining or improving their health rather than a performance of their race or gender politics. With the help of thriving online natural hair cultures and marketplaces, wellness and Black beauty discourses cut across national boundaries. Sheryl, 42, another natural hair entrepreneur in Los Angeles, clarifies, "Certainly that is a movement. It is a movement for change and acceptance of hair in all kinds of styles. I think it's a movement to women getting away from extra chemicals that you don't need when there are manageable ways to wear your hair and it's beautiful."

A central concern for wellness and environmentalism separates the ways Black women discuss "naturalness" from narrower, texture-based definitions of the twentieth century, when "natural" simply denoted a short, cropped, Afro hairstyle. Now, women use the term "natural" not only to describe a wide range of hairstyles that leave kinky hair unstraightened, but also to describe the quality and character of the goods used to care for one's hair.

Participants in the natural hair movement use neoliberal biomedical logics to frame natural hair as a healthy consumer choice to avoid chemicals, use products with fewer preservatives, and wear hairstyles that permit more physically active lifestyles. Entrepreneurs like Sheila and Sheryl have created entire careers importing raw shea butter from West Africa and crafting organic concoctions to sell to women in their local communities. Through a broader conceptualization of "naturalness," Black women are marketing a hair politics that goes beyond a cultural aesthetic to incorporate wellness.

Black Women, Hair Politics, and Environmental Risk

Environmental justice advocates and ecofeminists have extensively critiqued the environmental movement for centering white, middle-class men's concerns.[3] Unfortunately, both ecofeminist and environmental justice frameworks tend to highlight one axis of identity at a time—either race *or* gender—obscuring or misrepresenting the experiences of people at the intersection of multiple categories of oppression. For example, the environmental justice movement's central critique is that poor communities and people of color have a long history of being ignored by environmental activists, academics, and policymakers, despite the fact that people of color and the poor bear an unequal burden of environmental hazards like pollution and toxic waste.[4] As Bryant and Mohai articulate, "To champion old growth forests or the protection of the snail darter or the habitat of spotted owls without championing clean safe urban environments or improved habitats for the homeless, does not bode well for future relations between environmentalists and people of color, and with the poor."[5] However, environmental justice activism has largely left out gender-specific concerns altogether.[6]

On the other hand, ecofeminists, through a form of cultural feminism, have argued that women's inherent, spiritual relationship with nature diverges from patriarchal capitalist imperatives to dominate and control the earth's resources. Ecofeminists importantly note that women suffer disproportionately from environmental risks, and that women are expected to serve as gatekeepers for their families' bodies against environmental toxins through the gendered social organization of responsibility during pregnancy and for feeding, caring, and shopping for their families.[7] However, by highlighting women's mystic connection to nature to support sustainable energy production and movements against militarism and corporatism, ecofeminism often essentializes and others women of color, particularly Indigenous and Black women, by upholding them as pre-civilized exemplars of a lifestyle mystically and naturally closer to the Earth.[8] In environmental activist discourses, as with many other social justice movements, all the minorities are men, all the modern women consumers are white, and women of color's unique environmental risk factors and experiences are ignored.

Environmental risk cannot be divorced from the postcolonial, Eurocentric, capitalist, and patriarchal cultural context in which women of color across the Black Atlantic live. While environmental feminists have recently piqued concerns about chemical toxicity in cosmetics and genetically modified organisms (GMOs), scholars, activists, and public health officials frequently fail to consider racial differences in women's beauty practices and the social hierarchies that produce these differences. Beauty myths pressure women of all races to approximate idealized and unattainable physical standards, but white-centered feminine beauty ideals more intensely compel Black women to discipline their bodies. As legal scholar Devon Carbado explains, "precisely because Black women have historically been masculinized, they have had to expend more energy and resources quite literally making themselves up as women."[9] Overall, Black women apply cosmetic products that, when tested, contain higher levels of carcinogenic chemicals like formaldehyde and synthetic hormones than products used by the general population.[10] Straightening systems like chemical relaxers, Brazilian blowouts, and keratin treatments are the main culprits. Such products adhere to the dominant feminine standard of beauty that valorizes long, straight hair. While hair relaxer use among white women is rare, one study found that 95% of African American women surveyed under age 45 and 85% of women older than 45 used them.[11] Many African American women combine chemical relaxers with heat straightening, and heat is hypothesized to further facilitate penetration and absorption of carcinogenic chemicals into the body.[12]

Most consumers assume that if a product is on the shelf at a store, then it is safe. But unlike pharmaceutical drugs and food, cosmetic products are rarely subject to pre-market approval by regulatory bodies like the Food and Drug Administration (FDA). In the United States, cosmetics companies are not required to list fragrance or trade-secret ingredients in their order of predominance, as with other products.[13] As a result, issues with the healthiness of products tend to be handled through recalls, after products are already on shelves, have reached consumers, and a critical mass of consumers have experienced and reported physical harm. This is dangerous, because many chemicals and microtoxins in beauty products are more harmful when topically applied than when eaten, because the skin lacks a detoxifying mediator like the liver.[14] Research also suggests that chemicals like parabens in haircare products may affect the fetus in utero through their pregnant mothers.[15]

As a child, I never questioned if there was an alternative to the weeping sores I'd develop after my monthly relaxers. These sores would leave a sticky residue on my scalp that I simply endured until I washed and styled my hair the next week. Hair relaxers frequently cause scalp lesions like those I experienced, which users learn to accept as an unfortunate and temporary side effect. (And it turns out that chemicals are already more easily absorbed by the scalp than other areas of the body, like the forearm, palm, or abdomen). Both sodium hydroxide and calcium hydroxide, the two most used active ingredients in chemical relaxers, are also the active ingredients in many industrial solvents like brick and cement cleaners. Lisa, a 35-year-old woman in Los Angeles, reflected on her traumatic first relaxer treatment during our conversation: "I was like, 'it's burning!' and my stylist she was like, 'I haven't even gotten to the other side [of your head].' She put her hands on my head and came out with a whole chunk of my hair in her hand." Brie, a 35-year-old from Cape Town, recalled the pain and the pressure of hair straightening in our interview:

> I remember my first relaxer. I was like eight or nine already and since then it has been straight hair. It should be straight because it's nice it's more accepting, everyone else is doing it. Never mind the burns that you got and the hair loss and the breakage. And just having to sit through it.

Twenty-six-year-old Raven from Cape Town, shrugging, reflected on her mother's common justification for her monthly chemical burns: "Beauty is pain."

But beauty is much more than that. The lesions caused by chemical burns facilitate the entry of micro-toxins into the body that are linked to a wide range of reproductive issues.[16] The chemicals in haircare products interfere with the endocrine system, which is responsible for regulating human growth, development, and reproduction.[17] A study of more than 23,000 pre-menopausal African American women determined that the estrogen-mimicking phthalates used as fragrance in hair relaxers are linked to uterine fibroids, which affect Black women at two- to three-times higher rates than white women, and are the leading cause of hysterectomies in the United States.[18] The stakes are life itself. Another National Institutes of Health-funded study of a diverse group of 33,974 participants ages 34–75 found that ever using relaxers was associated with a significantly higher risk of uterine cancer, with frequent use carrying an even higher association with illness—an association not observed for other common hair processes like permanent, semipermanent, or temporary hair dyeing.[19]

When Corliss, a 62-year-old retiree in Charlotte, was pregnant with her first child, a fibroid tumor grew alongside and eventually overtook her unborn baby, forcing her to need cesarean sections for all three of her following pregnancies. She relaxed her hair from middle school until her early sixties. A 2012 study found that ever using hair relaxers, duration of use, frequency of use, and total number of burns incurred by hair relaxers were all positively associated with the risk of developing fibroid tumors.[20] Given that some women relax their children's hair at young ages with the help of "kiddie perms" marketed to toddlers and sold cheaply at most convenience stores, some girls have been exposed to toxins in chemical relaxers for a decade by the time they reach adolescence. Relaxing kinky hair is often treated as a rite of passage into Black womanhood and into the Black beauty shop—an historically and uniquely important site for fostering sisterhood among Black women.[21] Black beauty culture has inadvertently exacerbated Black women and girls' environmental risk.

Several other studies have hypothesized that chemicals commonly found in Black haircare products are linked to asthma, low birth weights, miscarriages, breast cancer, and early onset puberty—all of which Black women experience in higher than average numbers.[22] Estrogen and xenoestrogen hormones in parabens, which are used as preservatives in many personal care products, are also linked to higher rates and lethality of breast cancer among African American women.[23] These risks are exacerbated for Black hairstylists who encounter these chemicals daily.[24] In addition, products packaged for salons are not required to list ingredients and chemicals because the Fair Packaging Act, which regulates how consumer products are labeled and mandates that the contents and source of an item are transparently disclosed to buyers, does not apply to products used at professional establishments.[25] Fannie, a 45-year old hairstylist and traveling natural hair expert, expressed this concern in our interview, saying, "I would rather do natural hair. I know natural hair is in its natural state and you can do natural styles on it; you don't have to breathe in carcinogens." Even nonchemical alternatives like weaves or extensions can lead to serious scalp diseases like traction alopecia, so natural styles seem to be the healthiest option.[26]

In addition, a study of three hundred women in New York found that African American women who use hair products before age thirteen begin menstruating earlier, and that relaxers were particularly linked to early menstruation.[27] Some Black girls show signs of puberty as young as age *two*, and Tiwary observed that African American girls' premature sexual development regressed when they discontinued use of hair-care products containing hormonally-active ingredients.[28] At a meeting about Black hair and health at the 2016 Nappywood Festival in Los Angeles, Black Women for Wellness program manager Nourbese Flint urged attendees to consider, "What does it mean when little Black girls look older than they are and we are already hypersexualized?" Flint's comment suggests that relaxers are technologies of biopower that reinforce controlling images of Black women as hot mommas and jezebels, which are "designed to make racism, sexism, and poverty appear to be natural, normal, and an inevitable part of everyday life."[29]

Hair straightening is perhaps further to blame for racial health disparities because it discourages physical activity. Straight hair precludes many women's ability to be physically active, since sweat and water revert chemically and thermally straightened hair to its natural texture. A recent study by public health researchers found that Black adolescent girls (ages fourteen to seventeen) may avoid exercise because they feared their hair becoming "nappy" due to sweat.[30] Janine, a 36-year-old television executive living in California, told me, the "only reason why I'm not going to train for a triathlon was my hair." Janine's feeling is common.

In 2011, former US Surgeon General Regina Benjamin suggested hair maintenance was a main deterrent from exercising for Black women, as the slightest moisture from perspiration can ruin a style that takes time, money, and effort to attain.[31] Correspondingly, African Americans' rates of obesity, heart disease, diabetes, and cancer are higher than any other racial group in the United States.[32] After controlling for age, African American women are almost twice as likely to be diagnosed with diabetes than non-Hispanic whites.[33] Even though regulatory neglect, white-centered beauty norms, and Black beauty culture put Black women's health at such severe risk, popular discourse regarding the relationship between Black women's beauty practices and their health outcomes has been almost nonexistent—until recently.

(Bio)medicalizing Black Hair

In 2009, comedian Chris Rock's documentary *Good Hair* sparked a global conversation about the politics of Black hair by exploring the toll that hair straightening takes on Black women's emotional, physical, and financial health as they endeavor to meet white-centric standards for beauty and appearance.[34] Some of the focus of *Good Hair* was not new. Opponents of chemical hair relaxers have long critiqued Black women's styling choices using cultural arguments. Most prominently, the Black Power Movement in the United States and the Black Consciousness Movement in South Africa portrayed natural hair as one way for individuals to aesthetically embrace their African cultural heritage. But in a new and powerful strategy for confronting the relaxer's social power, *Good Hair* constructed chemical relaxing as a medical health issue through scientific demonstration. In one scene, Rock meets with a chemist to learn about sodium hydroxide—often referred to as "lye"—the main active ingredient in most chemical hair relaxers. Sporting a white lab coat and thick protective goggles in front of a massive backdrop of the periodic table of elements, the "chemical genius" explains that relaxers work to straighten hair by breaking down the protein bonds that create hair's curl pattern. In the scene, the chemist demonstrates how sodium hydroxide can eat through the flesh of a chicken cutlet. Like a cooking show, the cameras then pan to three beakers with aluminum soda cans soaking in sodium hydroxide to represent the chemical's impact over time. At one hour, the metal can has become transparent, at two hours it is liquefying, and by four hours the can has completely disintegrated. The time-lapse demonstration grotesquely mirrors the way Black women commonly extend relaxers' application time, sometimes fighting through chemical burns, in hopes of getting their hair as straight as possible.

The scientific framing in this scene proved a powerful pedagogical tool, and the film's popularity seemed to raise the environmental consciousness of many women of African descent around the world. Dozens of interviewees referenced the film in our conversations about their understanding of natural hair in the 2010s. The impact was so vast that even those who did not actually watch it felt its impact. For example, Krystal reflected:

> I don't remember seeing Afros or twist-outs until I was in my junior or senior year of college [2009–2011]. I remember the movie *Good Hair* by Chris Rock coming out and that steered me to not go back to my relaxer. And I didn't even see the movie. I've never seen the movie to this day. I just remember seeing previews of it. The talk around it really got people to say hey, we don't need that.

While *Good Hair* never explicitly presents natural hair or naturalness as a solution, it is probably no coincidence that the film's debut coincided with the rebirth a new and qualitatively unique way of thinking about Black haircare in the twenty-first century.

Warnings that chemical relaxers are both physically and psychologically dangerous proliferated in Black women's online blogs and vlogs in the 2010s, such that many Black women began to understand physical ailments as direct results from years of chemical straightening.[35] *Creamy crack*, a colloquial euphemism referring to some women's obsessive, drug-like dependence on chemical relaxers, took on new significance when viewed through a public health lens. In an article about online natural hair communities, Gill asserts that "allusions to the highly addictive crack cocaine and the destruction it has wrought in Black communities is intentional and highlights what many Black women feel is at stake in twenty-first century conversations about Black hair."[36] Transitioning to natural hair and natural haircare is a way for some Black women to avoid what they now see as a pathological reliance on dangerous consumer products.

As Black women began to view chemicals as the source of danger and harm, natural hair movement spaces projected nature as a wholesome and healing alternative. The idea that chemicals are just as responsible for Black women's pain as the cultural idealization of straight hair necessitates a solution that incorporates both transitions to natural hair textures *and* changes in the quality of Black haircare products. Natural hair influencers widely construct natural hair as a healthy choice by describing their natural hair journeys as transitions from illness to wellness. Bloggers' first-person testimonials ground the information they distribute in their embodied, lived experiences of transformation. Whitney White (@Naptural85) is perhaps the most popular natural hair blogger, with over 1.24 million YouTube subscribers and 715,000 Instagram followers. As a social media influencer whose presence dates to 2009, White's example of framing Black hair struggles in health terms has undoubtedly shaped the trajectory of the natural hair movement. Not only do White's vlog tutorials instruct viewers on how to evaluate the toxicity of ingredients in consumer products, but they also suggest DIY organic alternatives to commercial products. The video demonstrating her signature flaxseed gel alone has attracted 1.4 million views. She uses phrases like "protein sensitive" and attributes her ability to grow long hair to having overcome struggles with fungal overgrowth, postpartum shedding, and anxiety. In her video "Why Your Hair Texture is Changing + Falling Out: My Detailed Story," White sits in what looks to be her bedroom, looking directly into the camera confessional-style, creating a feeling of intimacy with the viewer. She tells a sixteen-minute story about managing her vitamin deficiency, celiac disease, alopecia, candida overgrowth, adrenal fatigue, and how each health concern manifested outwardly in her appearance. Her videos advance the notion that Black women's bodies are worthy environments of care in their entirety, and that hair and health are intimately intertwined. White's long, thick, kinky hair and extensive vlog archive grounds the advice she gives in her visible transformation.

At in-person events like the Taliah Waajid World Natural Hair Show, Nappywood, and International Natural Hair Meetup Day, organizers link haircare and healthcare as forms of resistance against the backdrop of relaxers' known effects on the body. For example, during a natural hair event in South Los Angeles, a group of fifty women gathered in a private room at the back of a Mexican restaurant. Attendees snacked on chips and dip at long banquet tables while the organizer, lovingly nicknamed "Madame President" by this close-knit group of women, stood at the front of the room with an easel and a chart about hair porosity, pH balance, and chemicals to avoid. Madame President demonstrated how to create a two-strand twist hairstyle from start to finish using a model chosen from the audience. With dripping hands, she held up a jar of soupy, translucent virgin coconut oil. "Put this on your hair before you shampoo, maybe even leave it overnight to make detangling easier. Especially if you have high porosity hair, you're going to want to use this when you're styling because it penetrates the hair shaft." She continued, "And when you're done, you know you can also use this with your partner during sex!" Madame President informed attendees that coconut oil's antifungal properties can serve as an alternative to commercial intimate lubricants. Then, she passed out purple sheets entitled "Curly Girls Need to Know More than Curls!" with a multiple-choice quiz to assess our comprehension: True or false? Normal vaginal pH is 3.8–4.5, slightly acidic—true. Vitamin E has been known to boost sexual hormones—true. Glycerin is the best ingredient in sexual lubes—false. Homemade natural vaginal soaps made by a Black woman entrepreneur who also makes products for natural hair were raffled off at the end of the event. This organization later began selling multicolored T-shirts with the tagline "Curls Detox: Not Required." The product description for the shirt elaborated that curls "don't need detoxing because they aren't toxic. We have cared for our curls with loving care and we are proclaiming they are fine the way they are." In these ways, this natural hair enthusiast and influencer explicitly projects natural hair as a project for self-love, self-care, and wellness.

Natural hair movement spaces like this have become hubs for collaborative partnerships with wellness advocates and nonprofits. For example, at Curly Girl Collective's 2016 CurlFest event in Brooklyn, NY, yoga instructors led attendees in an outdoor class on the green expanse of Prospect Park, encouraging physical fitness, movement, and

FIGURE 3.1. Attendees practice yoga at an outdoor natural hair festival. Author's photo.

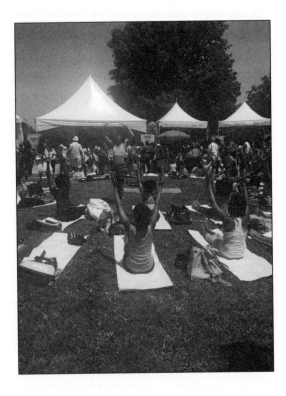

mindfulness. And across the country, health advocacy group Black Women for Wellness distributed informational pamphlets about hair relaxer toxicity at a natural hair meetup in Southern California. Their volunteers sat perched at booths alongside stands selling Africa-shaped earrings and T-shirts reading "All Natural No Lye." As Zina Saro-Wiwa likewise observes in an article for the New York Times, "[the natural hair] movement is characterized by self-discovery and health."[37]

Redefining "Good Hair" as "Healthy Hair"

In alignment with proliferating arguments that link hair care to over-all health, my interview data suggests that many Black women who go natural today do so as a wellness practice rather than, or in addition to, an outward political or fashion statement. Women I interviewed repeatedly told health recovery narratives in our discussions about their motivations for transitioning to natural hair. Many believed that their illnesses and those of other Black women they knew were the direct ramifications of their chemical relaxer use. My conversation with Olivia, a 32-year-old magazine editor and entrepreneur living in Brooklyn, NY is one such example. Olivia's relationship with her mother was central to her understanding of beauty because of the contrast between how her mother's cottony hair texture was regarded in her family and the jealous gazes Olivia's smooth silky curls attracted. Olivia's mother hated her own natural hair because her sisters had made fun of it since she was a child, calling it nappy and ugly. She considered Olivia's "good" biracial hair texture fit to avoid relaxers, but Olivia's relatively tight curl pattern to be socially unacceptable. "Good hair" and "bad hair" distinc-tions were hurtful for both women. The turning point in her family was her mother's failing health: "[My mom] permed [her hair] until she was diagnosed with breast cancer and she got a double mastectomy. Luckily, she didn't have to do chemo, but I think for obvious reasons there was a shift in her life . . . Why do we have to put all these chemicals in my scalp this is not healthy?" Olivia's mother did not choose natural hair as political resistance against white beauty norms, like many African American women in her age cohort had done in the 1960s and 1970s Black Is Beautiful era. Rather, she chose natural hair against a lifetime of emotional trauma and a broad societal devaluation of kinky hair upon thinking critically about relaxer's impact on her health. Olivia's family redefined "good hair" as healthy hair. Olivia's mother's motivation to transition to natural hair illustrates the power that reframing personal care choices in medical and environmental health terms can have in resisting colorism, racism, and deeply-internalized social stigma.

Like Olivia's mom, Michelle (49, Los Angeles) went natural in response to a developing illness. Michelle stopped chemically relaxing her hair a few months before we met in the parking lot of the Los Angeles Convention Center, both lost on our way to the 2015 Afrolicious Natural Hair Show. Michelle started relaxing her hair when she was eleven years old and continued to do so for the next three decades, accepting the monthly chemical burns as part of what it took to look presentable for her white-collar job. She transitioned to natural hair after finding out that she had dangerously high blood pressure. Her hypertension forced her to become more discerning about what she put in and on her body: "I just had to change my lifestyle and maybe about three or four years ago I started juicing a lot. Every day I do a green drink and a red drink. I try to stay away from anything that's really salty or sugary, just trying to maintain my health. Then I found out through maintaining my health that some of the things that I was juicing was also good for my hair." The dietary changes Michelle made increased her knowledge about a natural lifestyle's potential benefits to her appearance. She worked her way from blending shakes with spinach, turmeric, and kale to concocting do-it-yourself creams made with coconut oil, avocado oil, and honey for her hair. She noticed that avoiding parabens and sulfates caused the whites of her eyes brighten, her skin to clear, and her hair to grow faster. Michelle began reading natural hair blogs online for more recipes and now actively participates in natural hair meetups as a volunteer organizer.

Several other women I interviewed situated transitioning to natural hair and joining natural hair communities as part of a broad lifestyle shift to prioritize holistic wellness and self-care. Krystal (24, Tallahassee) explained:

> Even my products are organic and that actually drew me into [natural hair]. I don't think one causes the other but I think it's connected. It's bringing awareness of the other. The natural is bringing awareness to the green movement. When someone is a natural it's kind of like okay, you're a natural, so why not be all the way natural? Why not be green?

Likewise, Evelyn (42, Johannesburg), an entrepreneur, told me:

> Healthy eating was important before, but more so after I went natural because I was researching all of these ingredients about keeping your body healthy and how to grow long hair and then that you learn you are supposed to keep your balance of water to hydrate and to exercise. All of that kind of stuff. Eat healthy food and take a multivitamin if you need to. It mattered more when I started growing my hair natural and my first goal was to have healthy hair that actually grows.

Brie (35, Cape Town) held a similar view, elucidating, "Literally the most profound 'aha' moment is the fact that I started transitioning with my hair but it's been a transition overall. My skin, oh my god. It started with my hair but now it's how I feed my body and changing the way I eat. Embracing more natural things in my body. I've also joined a gym." Lauren (26, Brooklyn) also witnessed a transformation from illness to wellness after adopting an ethos of naturalness. When Lauren became a caretaker for her former romantic partner's ill mother, she observed how much the woman benefitted from ensuring food was chemically safe by juicing at home: "She was on a strict diet, so we had to juice for her and I just started learning about it and watching documentaries. I just became obsessed with it and I saw the benefits because she *glowed*."

This inspired Lauren to do a total body detox as a preventative measure, which encompassed changes to her diet, haircare regimen, and contraceptive preferences. She continued juicing, got off the Depo birth control shot, and shaved her head. Lauren told me, "I cut my hair. I wanted the chemicals out of my hair. I had to get the chemicals out of me and I have to start caring more about everything that I'm putting into my body." Lauren noticed that her migraines and depression both receded, and she now aspires to transition from her career in waitressing to establishing her own juice truck so that she can share her transformative health experience with others.

Xena (25, Minneapolis) stumbled upon natural hair websites around 2012. There, she discovered that the styling products she used to care for her curly hair contained carcinogenic chemicals and that flat ironing her hair straight daily with temperatures up to four hundred degrees Fahrenheit was detrimental to its health. Xena began mixing recipes from YouTube in her kitchen using coconut oil, castor oil, and natural essential oils like tea tree and rosehip seed—and she saw her curls thrive. She began a journey into holistic wellness and eventually trained to become a reiki master. A self-described *bruja*, her apartment, which doubles as her reiki clinic, is packed with crystals, lit by Himalayan salt lamps, and filled with the scent of burning palo santo wood. Transitioning to natural haircare prompted a qualitative change that reorganized Xena's sense of self as well as her understanding of what it meant to care for her and her clients' bodies. Several other women I interviewed have pursued occupations around natural care and wellness upon transitioning to natural hair. Anita (47, Los Angeles) became a professional advocate for breastfeeding in Black communities, and Zaire (24, Inglewood) went back to school to study nutrition upon joining natural hair communities online. Just as styling curly hair straight requires that one align her lifestyle accordingly—by avoiding rain and sweating, for example—adopting an ethos of naturalness seems to affect how Black women think about a wide range of lifestyle practices.

That many Black women have transitioned to natural hair to mitigate the threat of illness or actively pursue wellness demands that they get to know their bodies' needs in new and intimate ways. Each of these women monitored anew how their bodies looked, performed, healed, and felt as they engaged in conscious care for themselves and others. Their stories of commitment to natural remedies are grounded in an embodied experience of transformation from illness to wellness. While the central emphasis on health in these hair testimonies may not sound overtly political or activist, I argue that the way these women deploy natural hair remains a strong expression of Black feminist thought. As Collins posits, Black feminism is grounded in Black women's standpoints, or situated, experienced-based understandings, and is reflected in ordinary Black women's expressions of self-determination.[38] By overcoming externally defined white-centric standards for feminine beauty that compel Black women to enact violence upon their own bodies, these women's transitions to natural hair are radical practices of self-valuation. Like Saro-Wiwa explained in her piece for the *New York Times*, "whether transitioners believe it or not, demonstrating this level of self-acceptance represents a powerful evolution in political expression."[39] Viewing the Black female body as an environment worthy of protection and care is just as radical as the Black Nationalist goal of economic redistribution. After all, groups are unable to take advantage of redistributed material resources if they are ill, unable to reproduce, or no longer alive. As Audre Lorde so powerfully declared, "caring for myself is not self-indulgence, it is self-preservation, and that is an act of political warfare."[40]

Sociologists theorize the phenomenona of redefining social problems as medical conditions as *medicalization* and the commodification of health problems as *biomedicalization*.[41] Bolstered with the power and authority of medicine, scientists and doctors increasingly offer and promote new types of surgeries, pills, enhancements, and chemical processes to patient-consumers as solutions for human experiences, like desire or humiliation, by constructing bodies as defective sources. Scholars have widely documented the medicalization and biomedicalization of beauty, observing that women are expected to turn to medical procedures (i.e., cosmetic surgery) to satisfy and alleviate low self-esteem and body image concerns.[42] The domain of medicine increasingly extends to healthy, "normal" bodies as well. Biomedicalization explains the rising preoccupation with wellness in our postmodern, neoliberal era, where health has become a commodity and a signifier of a person's ability to responsibly self-manage. With contemporary shifts toward unrestrained markets, privatization, and the decline in social welfare in the name of individualism, people, not unlike the market itself, are increasingly considered privately-responsible for the costs of social reproduction and economic success.[43] The neoliberal idea of the self-as-project constructs women as both subjects and consumers who must take on "appropriate" consumption practices, creating a culture of self-scrutiny in which women engage in self-surveillance, self-monitoring, and self-disciplining.[44] For example, Berkowitz theorizes the popularization of Botox as the biomedicalization of aging, and predicts that a lack of wrinkles will come to signify wealth and class status in the near future, much like dental health already does.[45]

Medical and biomedical frames tend to depoliticize social issues by locating the source of a problem in an individual's private body and the solution to a problem in the consumer market, instead of focusing on structural and cultural dynamics. For example, Kaw's study of trends in Asian American women's experiences with cosmetic surgery finds that the medical industry subtly perpetuates white-centric beauty standards by encouraging Asian American women to select procedures that obscure their phenotypical racial markers, rather than critiquing the effects of European colonization and military occupation, Western hegemony, and global white supremacy.[46] Likewise, Kauer describes how the neoliberal wellness model that idealizes slim, white, "fit" bodies in popular Western representations of yoga operates to serve the weight loss, fitness, and pharmaceutical industries rather than honor yoga's roots in Indian physical, mental, and spiritual practices. Kauer points to popular sexualized and commodified media images of white women that saturate women's magazines and the yoga industry more broadly as obfuscating a necessary discussion about the barriers to adequate healthcare, safe spaces for meditation, and affordable training that many people of color, LGBT communities, and poor folks face despite the fact that they endure higher rates of stress. She argues that these exclusionary images pathologize queer and fat bodies, as well as empty yoga of its potential for spiritual and feminist transformation.[47] Discourses within the natural hair movement depart from this trend by starting with a critique of gendered racial inequality and deploying the authority of scientists to suggest naturalness, rather than intervention, as a more ethical and socially just alternative. For instance, cosmetic chemist-turned-entrepreneur Erica Douglas, who also goes by the moniker Sister Scientist, tours natural hair festivals and the natural hair blogosphere in her white lab coat discussing the importance of avoiding the phthalates and carcinogens that disproportionately appear in products for Black women. Likewise, health scientist Audrey Davis-Sivasothy is widely sought after to speak on her books *The Science of Black Hair* (2011), *Hair Care Rehab* (2012), and *The Science of Transitioning* (2015) that subtly present a return to nature as a "cure" for damaged, processed hair.

This is not to say that the natural hair movement escapes an engagement with neoliberal consumer culture, or even that natural hair is hair that is left alone. A burgeoning flock of men and women have become natural hair entrepreneurs, concocting and selling products with organic ingredients to care for natural hair with descriptions like "sulfate-free" and "paraben-free." Contemporary advocates of natural hair view specialized haircare products as the key to unlocking more style choices for women of color, making commodification and consumerism central to contemporary organizing around natural hair. For example, new services like Mayavana, owned by Black beauty and technology company Techturized, analyze clients' hair strands under a microscope to scientifically recommend the "perfect" customized products by hair porosity, diameter, and elasticity. Furthermore, the newly emergent natural hair show caters toward the lay *consumer*, unlike traditional hair shows and

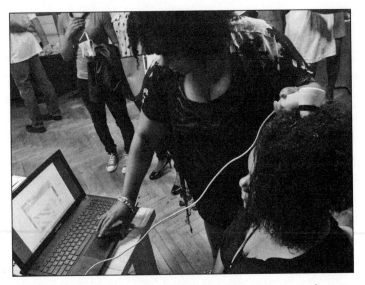

FIGURE 3.2. Scientist studies woman's hair under a microscope for custom product recommendations. Author's photo.

beauty conventions that are primarily attended by industry profession-als. At a typical natural hair show, business owners pitch their products to women who come and go from their booths, while panels of "experts" including beauty bloggers, hairstylists, and specialists like Sister Scien-tist host discussions on healthy hair maintenance regimens and perform styling demonstrations on guests. Black hair historians Ayana Byrd and Lori Tharps call these actors "naturalpreneurs."[48] Broadly, naturalpre-neurs argue that natural hair is healthy and beautiful by promoting products that claim to define curls, lessen frizz, detangle, and increase manageability without using harmful chemicals, both in-person at hair events and online through product reviews on blogs.

Selling Intersectional Wellness

Many naturalpreneurs see themselves as not only business owners, but also as intersectional environmental justice advocates intervening in a racist, sexist, and toxic consumer market that ignores Black women's specific needs. They engage in what Mackendrick calls the "precautionary consumption"—the practice of evaluating the toxicity of ingredients in food, cleaning, and cosmetic purchases.[49] In response to increasing consciousness about the health risks of relaxers, natural hair communities likewise advocate for cautious consumption of natural products as responsible, ethical, healthful, and necessary. However, unlike their white, middle-class counterparts, Black women routinely find themselves ignored by an organic personal care market that assumes a white subject. On one hand, the ethnic haircare aisle is disproportionately toxic; on the other hand, organic options are often naively colorblind. Natural hair shows and individual naturalpreneurs work to fill that gap.

Stacey (29, Cape Town), a cosmetics entrepreneur, brought up this issue during our conversation. I met Stacey at her shop in a market under a train station in Observatory, a predominantly Black and Coloured[50] neighborhood. Here, she sells her line of natural hair and body salves alongside a Rastafarian barbershop and a woman vending vintage clothes. She initially began mixing her hair- and skincare products at home because her son's newborn skin was too sensitive for the commercial products available at her local convenience store. Later, Stacey began selling her at-home mixtures to fill a gap she saw in the market: "I do what I do for Black women . . . I don't feel like there is enough out here for us." Her best seller is a hair and body moisturizing milk, a simple, three-ingredient product made with aloe, a plant that grows wild throughout the Western Cape, olive oil, and natural lecithin. Like many other environmentalists of color, she openly separates herself from the traditional, mainstream environmental movement:

> They do all these things with the environment but they don't know how to deal with these Black people over here. "I don't want to have this conversation." Walk into the Clicks [a pharmacy chain in South Africa] aisle for our hair, it is relaxing hair products, coloring hair products. Nothing is literally good for you. Here is a group of women, and when I say women,

I take it for granted that I mean Black women, trans Black women, this umbrella of people that no one pays attention to.

Stacey elaborates that "in Cape Town, things that are natural are still marketed to white people, middle-class, and upper-class people with all this money. These people who are light and love and eat lentils and don't do harm to animals. All these beautiful things but they just don't deal with race." Her comments present both a structural critique of product availability in mainstream convenience stores and a cultural critique of the green consumer niche's privileged ignorance of Black women's needs. In short, an environmental consciousness is simply not enough for many Black women to make more healthful choices. Natural hair entrepreneurs fill gaps caused by regulatory neglect and eurocentrism in the green consumer industry by providing alternatives that serve natural-textured curly and kinky hair with natural ingredients.

Stacey actively prioritizes her peers as an underserved market by advertising her products in a Cape Town natural hair Facebook support group, by vending at natural hair festivals, and by opting for farmer's markets in Black and Coloured communities over big distribution deals with national retailers. Other natural hair entrepreneurs spread environmental consciousness by teaching Black women how to evaluate the toxicity of their haircare products. Sheila (45, Johannesburg), the woman I introduced at the start of this chapter, views her business as a platform for environmental education. She explained:

I really feel that people don't know not because they don't want to know but because nobody is there to educate, so I really want to, even in making my products, I ensure that I use conscious ingredients. If it is not certified organic, if it is not certified by ECOSET I don't use it. For me it is important. And also—the sustainability of it. If we take it from somewhere and the tree is becoming extinct then we can't use it. How is it sourced? You look at those little things before you even try and use the product. If it is taken from a country, who are they getting it from? Are people there enslaved to get the product? Every single ingredient that goes in there it is consciously sourced, it is a conscious product and when you use it, it is biodegradable. I'm able to educate and buying the product becomes the last thing I do after I've educated. You consciously buy because you understand what you buy.

Sheila makes her products with crops indigenous to Southern Africa, like mongongo oil and baobab oil. Everything she sells is sourced from Fair Trade and Community Trade initiatives, and nothing contains alcohol, parabens, sulfates, mineral oil, or ingredients tested on animals. Entrepreneur Sheryl (42, Los Angeles), similarly told me, "Even though a lot of those better ingredients are more expensive, we're going to have to cut our profits a little bit more to make sure that we care about this world, the state of health of the world." Her company also uses recyclable and biodegradable packaging. For these business owners, selling natural haircare products is the starting place of a broader intersectional politics. Beyond catering to a natural aesthetic, their goals include other issues that affect marginalized communities, like the burdens of toxic waste, capitalist imperialism, and slavery. Like other activists operating outside of the mainstream environmental movement, Sheila and Sheryl have "begun to shift the definition of environmentalism away from the exclusive focus on consumption to the sphere of work and production."[51]

Black women are frequently left out of dominant histories of environmental and gender-based activism because they haven't always labeled their work feminist—let alone ecofeminist—and face different issues than those with race and/or gender privilege.[52] For example, many Black women in the US women's movement eschewed feminism or opted for the label "womanist" to emphasize how race and class intersect to shape Black women's experience of gender.[53] Moreover, women of color often lack the resources to express their politics in privileged spaces, adding to their marginalization from dominant activist and academic discourses.[54] But viewing Black women's ideological and advocacy work within the natural hair movement as intersectional environmental feminism decenters environmental and feminist histories that exclusively empha-size the experiences, methods, and strategies of privileged groups. While not all these influencers identify as feminist, womanist, or environmen-talists, their deployment of naturalness is intersectional and political in effect. These naturalpreneurs have been in the forefront of the effort to create affordable, accessible, consciously-sourced cosmetic products.

Neoliberal Naturalness as Gendered Racial Formation

The natural hair movement's biomedicalized deployment of "natural-ness" reshapes how Blackness is managed, represented, and configured more broadly. White supremacist ideologies have repeatedly racialized Black bodies as closer to nature to legitimate Black people's position at the bottom of racial hierarchies.[55] A Western logic of oppositional nature-culture dualism has helped construct whiteness as the counter-image of Blackness, where Blacks are disorderly, chaotic, and wild and whites are rational, culturally superior, civilizing forces.[56] By associat-ing Black bodies with nature, whites justify their supposed imperatives to conquer, control, subjugate, and discipline Black bodies and nature at the same time. This racial project has been deeply gendered. Colo-nizers, slavers, scientists, and politicians alike have portrayed the Black female body as the essence of feminine primitiveness in a series of racial representations over the last five hundred years. As bell hooks and Cor-nel West point out, "from slavery to the present day, the Black female body has been seen in Western eyes as the quintessential symbol of a 'natural' female presence that is organic, closer to nature, animalistic, primitive."[57]

Sarah Baartman's story is perhaps the most powerful example of the racialization of Black women's bodies as inferior through associa-tions with a supposedly primitive nature. Born in the Gamtoos Valley in South Africa, Baartman was sold to a British doctor and became known as the "Hottentot Venus" because of her caged exhibition in freak shows throughout nineteenth-century Europe. Baartman's naked body, particularly her posterior, drew gaping spectators from near and far in what Rosemarie Garland-Thomson calls "inverted, parodic beauty pageants."[58] A series of white captors exploited her body for financial gain, "scientifically" defining Black bodies as deviant, hypersexual, and subhuman in the process. In their biography of Baartman's life, Crais and Scully argue that the spectacle of the Hottentot Venus "confirmed the inequality and unfitness of all women, for women were closer to nature, and the Hottentot Venus was the closest of them all."[59] Onlookers gazed at Baartman's dark body "not as a human being but as an extraordinary object of nature existing at the edge of the exotic and grotesque."[60] Associating Baartman's body with nature served to legitimize racial inequality between Europeans and Africans, and especially between Black women and white women.[61]

Similarly, slaveholders in the American South invoked gendered associations between Blackness and nature through stereotypes about Black women's unbridled sexuality and natural propensity for childbirth.[62] Black women were projected as bestial to rationalize the most intimate forms of servitude, exploitation, and dehumanization. This enabled slaveholders to justify rape and the use of Black women as chattel breeders and wet nurses for their own children.[63] The white elite in the United States viewed breastfeeding as animalistic, so "breeder" enslaved women were forced to breastfeed their mistresses' babies, often before or instead of feeding their own children. My interviewee Anita (47, Los Angeles), who is both a professional breastfeeding advocate and a natural hair event organizer in Southern California, explained to me that this contributed to the malnourishment and death of many enslaved Black children and forms the basis of continuing stigmas against breastfeeding in Black communities. In the twentieth century, the US government deployed parallel discourses about Black women's bodies through tropes like the incessantly-breeding "welfare queen" that blame poor Black women for their marginalized political, economic, and social positions.[64] Discourses depicting Black women as uncivilized and needing to be tamed have also been used to justify forced sterilizations and other coercive birth control schemes.[65] Heller notes that even left-leaning ecologists evoke racist and sexist tropes about Black women's nearness to nature to accuse poor women of color of using up too much of Earth's resources by "overpopulating."[66] By reducing Black women to either a source of labor or a social burden, each of these examples operates as a gendered racial project that explains away unequal material relationships in white supremacist patriarchal and capitalist society. Black women confront these essentialist understandings about their "exotic naturalness" when they return to natural hairstyles, especially because stigmas that Black women are wild and undisciplined have been mapped onto kinky and curly hair textures.[67] Recall, this is precisely why Black beauty culturists of the twentieth century linked respectability to straight hair as a racial uplift strategy.

In her essay on eco-womanism, Riley points out that "because of the historical and current treatment of Blacks in dominant Western ideology, Black womanists must confront the dilemma of whether we should strive to sever or reinforce the traditional association of Black people with nature that exists in dominant Western thought."[68] The natural hair movement decisively takes a position. Drawing on Black feminist and environmentalist themes, the natural hair movement *rearticulates* associations between Black women's bodies and nature, infusing them with new political meaning by centering Black women's subjectivity, giving rise to new and distinct political meanings. Influencers and businesses like Naptural85, Madame President, Mayavana, Sister Scientist, and my interviewee Sheila reclaim colonial narratives and revise pejorative associations between Black women and nature by linking natural hair with intersectional wellness ideologies and foregrounding Black women's embodied experiences of illness and transformation. Instead of signifying wildness, laziness, or backwardness, contemporary natural hair politics disseminates counterhegemonic discourses that naturalness is a healthy, progressive, and responsible choice that questions an increasingly-passé authority polluting its way to environmental doom—all marketable qualities in the 2010s and early 2020s. Black women with natural hair

increasingly see themselves and are read by others as discerning, politically "woke" consumers. Furthermore, Black women's demand for
natural products and the resulting explosion of entrepreneurship has
positioned Black women as leading authorities in the green consumer
industry. Whereas proximity to naturalness was used by whites to deny
Black women's access to citizenship in the seventeenth, eighteenth,
nineteenth, and twentieth centuries, natural hair politics harnesses
naturalness to align modern Black femininity with twenty-first-century
neoliberal understandings of good citizenship.

Dilemmas in Natural Consumer Politics

As other feminist scholars of the body have argued, the biomedicalization of health and bodywork under neoliberalism tends to stratify along
class dimensions.[69] Consumerism and class are often tangled up with
exercising "wokeness," displaying good citizenship, participating in natural hair culture, and avoiding the trap of toxic haircare practices. Just as
smooth skin, white teeth, and toned bodies are increasingly made possible by access to commodified technologies, services, and products, so
too are many natural solutions for natural hair. Likewise, contemporary
natural hair politics is both constrained and enabled by its entanglement
with capitalism and consumer culture. Krystal describes the transformative opportunities consumerism has provided her: "Due to the plethora
of products, women are making a more personal choice because they are
available. I can make a personal choice to deal with who I am at my core
if I want to and I'm going to have the resources to do so."

However, instead of being "creamy crack" addicts to hair relaxers,
natural hair communities can create "product junkies" who amass an
ever-growing supply of natural hair products in search of a regimen they
feel works well enough to achieve their styling goals. "Product junkie"
has become a widespread colloquialism in natural hair communities
and an expected stage for new naturalistas as they endeavor to discover
what works for them. My conversations in the field typically began with

compliments on my hair, followed by the pointed inquiry, "What do you *use*?" Given that I accumulated a multitude of free samples from attending hair events weekly, I tended to apply a medley of whatever I had on hand at home and failed to have sufficient answers to give my interviewees. In one memorable instance, a beauty blogger waved me over and requested to feature me on her website. During the interview, she pressured me to reveal a favorite "must-have" product and became frustrated when I could not. This emphasis on commodification and consumer culture makes sense in the current neoliberal context, where "rights-based political movements multiply as disenfranchised individuals and groups use the technologies, processes, and subjectivities of consumer culture to achieve their goals."[70]

Tatiana, the founder of an international natural hair event, told me that her main tasks were securing and distributing samples of healthy hair products to local hosts around the world. Advertisements of giveaway SWAG (stuff we all get) bags filled with packets of shampoos and creams serve as incentives for thousands of eventgoers to show up in person, rather than participate in natural hair forum discussions and advocacy exclusively online. At a natural hair event in Brooklyn, New York, thousands of women formed a snaking line around Prospect Park, waiting for hours to receive a first-come first-served VIP product gift set. These women had no idea what would be included in the bags and were content to wait patiently as stations for food, music, and dancing buzzed just beyond.

The emphasis on consumerism in natural hair spaces makes sense in today's neoliberal moment. All racial projects are grounded in social structures and ideologies of specific moments and places, and neoliberal culture is central to the forms of surveillance, control, and resistance that manifest in the early twenty-first century. Neoliberalism idealizes "self-managing, autonomous[,] and enterprising" subjects.[71] In this postindustrial order, the body is a signifier of discipline and good citizenship, requiring that individuals interact with consumer capitalism to demonstrate moral worth.[72]

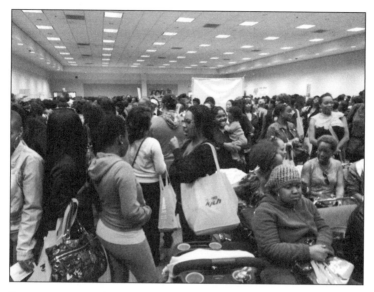

FIGURE 3.3. Attendees carry totes filled with free SWAG (stuff we all get) at a natural hair festival. Author's photo.

Many scholars argue that the neoliberal rhetoric of individual choice, entitlement and pleasure depoliticize social justice issues by grounding citizenship in consumption.[73] Others likewise assert that neoliberal politics minimally disrupts structural race, class, and gender inequality by empowering individual women at best, and reproducing social hierarchies at worst.[74] Feminist anti-beauty scholars fall in this camp, viewing beauty culture's capitalist engine as driving and depleting women's subjectivities.[75] In their assessment, beauty is a disciplinary force, a form of power that systematically subjugates women. For example, Naomi Wolf argues that while the women's movement of the 1970s successfully deconstructed most fictions of femininity like domesticity, motherhood, and chastity, "beauty myths" remained intact.[76] Like Wolf, Faludi argues that women paradoxically face increasing pressures to be thin, young, and demure despite gains in political, sexual, and economic power and self-determination.[77] These scholars believe that strengthening and all-encompassing beauty ideals are rooted in and maintained by corporations that rely on women as consumers who seek to embody them. Elias, Gill, and Scharff that argue under neoliberalism, all women are expected to engage in "aesthetic entrepreneurship" due to the rising numbers of images and technologies to alter the way we look.[78]

Even as Black women spend greater percentages of their income on beautification,[79] partaking in "green" naturalness is not equally accessible to all. Many Black communities in the United States and across the Black Atlantic continue to exist in food deserts where organic produce and products for natural hair are unavailable or more expensive than in middle-class neighborhoods. Evelyn (42, Johannesburg) traveled across town to a health food store at an affluent mall in Sandton to find coconut oil and shea butter, which she had discovered were healthy products for use on natural hair after reading about them on blogs. She acknowledged, "It's harder if you don't have much to spend." We discussed affordability and food deserts further in our interview:

> JOHNSON: It is often the same thing in African American communities. It is mostly middle-class Black American communities who have access to this whole natural hair world as bloggers are creating it. It seems pretty similar [in South Africa].
>
> EVELYN: Same here. Just across the road is Alexander, and Alexander is actually near Sandton and the community is so, so, so bad, so sad. The food there is shit. It is not healthy at all. I wouldn't just buy food there especially because I now know. It's very cheap but it's what they can afford. Pick n Pay there is different from Pick n Pay here. There are two different worlds. The income disparities are so, so, so different. There's a big margin between the haves and the have nots . . . There are now a few Blacks who have access to the middle class but most people don't have access to internet to make conscious decisions about what they are going to eat to have choice. Some people are just concerned about filling their tummies, which is surviving. The thing is with poverty is it limits your options.

The privilege of choice is not available to many people of African descent living in the United States, and even fewer communities of African descent living in less-developed countries with more recent histories of state-sanctioned racial, economic, and spatial segregation, like during apartheid in South Africa just two decades ago.

But the pressure to purchase and procure expensive, healthy products remains, especially because many women have little knowledge about caring for their natural hair, and so they turn to the market for solutions. Raven (26, Cape Town) explained, "Because it is fairly new, women try every product that they can. Being natural has become an expensive movement. The first thing my friend said is where did you buy your product and I told her and she said this is three times as much as my normal product. For some people, you don't have a choice but to end up blowing out your hair." Corliss (62, Charlotte) aspires to act on her new environmental consciousness, but her financial situation deters her from doing so. She explained, "Because with my hair natural then I want to start using natural products, too. Right now, I have what I have and I'm going to use what I have because I'm money conscious." Brie (35, Cape Town) resented the pressure of consumerism in a natural hair Facebook group that she regularly participates in: "Sometimes the group, as much as it can be supportive, you can feel alienated because you don't follow that routine. I felt bad for not following that LOC method [a regimen that requires a separate liquid, oil, and cream product to style hair]. I'm a lazy natural and I don't do all of this."

Furthermore, because much of the biomedicalized discourse about natural hair begins and ends online, poor women and women in developing countries with natural hair are more likely to be read in their communities not as conscious or progressive consumers, but as unable to afford relatively-inexpensive relaxers. For example, the first thing Sheila (45, Johannesburg) did to symbolize her economic mobility when she got her first job was straighten her hair: "My first salary I went to relax my hair because for me, I was liberated. People need to see now that I can afford [getting my hair done]." Sheila acted based on the understanding that hair texture and styling mattered within her community, and that those around her would evaluate her character and achievements based on her ability to relax her hair. As her reflection illustrates, Black women engage in an ongoing dialogue about self, status, and society through their styling choices. Naturalness of the natural hair movement, then, is one aspect of producing and exercising a *middle-class* Black womanhood. Signifiers of economic security, ideal womanhood, and cultural competence are hugely dependent on context. While naturalness increasingly constructs a privileged, liberated body in middle-class communities, relaxed hair remains a signifier of economic distress in many working-class communities. An intersectional perspective that considers the interconnected and contextual nature of social systems shows that the natural hair movement can be both liberating for some Black women and non-existent for others, even if they share the same race and gender identities. In short, natural hair reveals as much about class as it does about race and gender.

Conclusion

Natural hair is understood differently in the twenty-first century than it was during the Black Is Beautiful crusade of the late 1960s. Then, the Afro primarily symbolized Black Power by rejecting white aesthetic standards and by celebrating a new Black cultural aesthetic. The new natural hair movement extends those goals through a broader deployment of the term "natural." As the health consequences of relaxer use became widely publicized, natural has come to describe both kinky or curly hair texture *and* the integrity of ingredients in haircare products and self-care practices. In other words, green is the new Black.

The second-wave feminist canon tends to suggest that any time and money women invest in beautification and aesthetics is wasteful, shallow, regressive, and oppressive, and that time women spend thinking about the external body is inherently about others—about attracting lovers, satisfying employers, triumphing over opposition, or appealing to social gatekeepers. However, critiques of consumer-based politics rarely involve immersion into the actual lives and motivations of those who, they argue, engage in coercive and depoliticized consumption. Such categorical evaluations of beauty culture collapse differences between local histories, cultures, and subjective experiences. Many women find identity and purpose through the processes of self-objectification and beauty consumerism, deriving gratification, creating bonds with one another, elevating causes, and exercising control over themselves and their environmental impact in the process.[80] As sociologist Raewyn Connell explains, "bodies may participate in disciplinary regimes not because they are docile, but because they are active."[81] This "subjective-aspect-within-being-as-object" must not be overlooked.[82] Empirically observing women in social life, especially through an intersectional lens attentive to differences in race, class, and culture, shows that beauty work can be both critical and political for those who have access to its tools. For if there is little doubt that neoliberal discourses of self-scrutiny and self-making echo across the world in the interest of global capitalism, the kind of subject being mobilized, the nature of self-making that is encouraged, the effects being produced, and their economic impacts cannot be assumed to be consistent. By taking seriously Black women's embodied experiences of pain, illness, pleasure, and comfort, natural hair has become more than the uniform of revolution. It is also an embodied and grassroots resistance against race, class, and gender health disparities, colorblindness within the growing green consumer industry, and governmental regulatory neglect of communities of color. This focus on health and wellness separates twenty-first-century natural hair politics from previous moments of Black beauty activism.

Everyday women's knowledge about their bodies is often dismissed or kept private, especially if they live in marginalized communities, are poor, or are of color. As the canonical feminist health text *Our Bodies, Ourselves* (1971) has demonstrated over the last fifty years, when real women share their embodied experiences, they inspire other women to improve their healthcare practices and catalyze radical movements at the community level. Natural hair movement influencers act as intersectional environmental activists by disseminating new practices that treat Black women's bodies as environments worthy of protection and that address the specific toxicity concerns Black women face. In doing so, they rearticulate stereotypical associations between Blackness and nature, constructing an ethos of naturalness and natural hair as progressive and healthful ways to care for the body. Some women overcome lifelong insecurities about their hair texture and are moved to resist external expectations for straight hair, suggesting that the authority of science and the power of biomedicalization can be harnessed from below in resistance against gendered racism. Though a reified relationship between Black women and nature has been beneficial for improving Black women's health awareness, options and outcomes in the current neoliberal era, like all racial projects, this relationship remains a social construction that is not universally stable, good, productive or free from co-optation. While biomedicalization can be a productive means for critiquing and undoing the emotional and embodied manifestations of race and gender oppression, it can simultaneously reproduce stratified class arrangements. Poor women, especially those in the Global South, have limited access to the discourses, products, and culture of natural wellness. So, racial projects do not only operate on racial systems; they have mutual implications for class and gender systems as well.

That many people are initially attracted to natural hair as a wellness choice and not as an outward political statement does not mean they do not come to see natural hair as having political implications or symbolism. Some naturalpreneurs I interviewed believe that the explosion in product development by Black women for women with coily hair is the best chance for redistributing economic power to Black beauty entrepreneurs and aesthetic power to people of African descent. Since the 1980s, the beauty supply market has operated and organized itself under white supremacist beauty ideals.[83] However, the natural hair movement's new aesthetic disrupts institutionalized racism and the exclusion of Black-owned businesses from the beauty supply industry as Black entrepreneurs monetize their experience caring for their own hair. Marcus, founder of an organization focused on advancing Black entrepreneurship in the beauty retail space, contemplated the influence of the natural hair movement on the beauty industry in our interview, vividly illustrating how Black beauty politics are mutually rooted in the discursive, the material, and the symbolic:

> I mean, the hair alone in Korean beauty supply stores—and remember there is 12,000 of them—the hair alone at the average Korean beauty supply store at any given time has about $150,000 worth of inventory on that wall for commercial hair. That's changing because of the fact that the hairstyle has gone natural . . . The problem is that [Korean business owners] don't want that to happen because when they sell a bundle of hair they make $30–40 off that bundle. And that's one bundle. When you sell a bottle of grease, and that's the natural product, you only make about $3–4. The Black-owned businesses welcome it because the one thing about the natural hairstyle, you know the natural movement, is that it happened outside of the box they are forcing.

However, white supremacy functions in multiple ways to destabilize Black women's attempts to maintain a Black-affirming and Black women-centered natural hair movement—through the control of resources and consumer orientations in the beauty industry, cultural appropriation, and texturism within Black communities—a topic I will discuss further in Chapter 5. Moreover, the experience of transitioning can be emotionally difficult, as Black women encounter a wide variety of responses to their natural hair as they navigate their lives. These reactions are also deeply important to what natural hair means in the twenty-first century.

4

Black Hair Matters

Beauty as Racial Protest

In early 2016, the United States presidential primary campaigns were in full swing. On February 23, Bernie Sanders and Hillary Clinton sat onstage before a racially-diverse group of citizens for a Democratic town hall in Columbia, South Carolina. Rather than debating one another, they held conversations with the crowd. A young Black woman, Kyla Gray, rose to pose a question to Senator Clinton during her hour-long session. Wearing a black top, glasses, and shoulder-length natural hair parted in the center and pulled back in a low puffy ponytail, Gray drew upon her recent experience "going natural" to push the presidential hopeful into a conversation about the growing anti-Black racism she noticed around her:

> Recently I stated wearing my hair natural and I've noticed the difference in the way some people address and look at me. In the wake of things like Ferguson and Black Lives Matter and the recent backlash against Beyoncé for her "Formation" video, there have been a lot of racial tensions recently in our nation. So, my question to you is: What do you intend to do to fix the broken racial tensions in our nation?[1]

The way Gray posed her question captures the *why* and *how* of Black beauty politics today. Like most women I interviewed, Gray does not suggest that she transitioned to natural hair for political reasons. Rather, she speaks of *noticing* a difference in how people saw and treated her as a Black woman with natural hair. Unlike during the Black Power era, when Afros were considered a tool for revaluating Afrocentric beauty, today women more often describe a process of politicization through the *experience* of transitioning to natural hair. Gray's question reveals that she came to view the treatment of her body—because of her natural hair—in racial terms and as an expression of broader racial tensions in the United States. Natural hair does not seem to be Gray's "uniform of rebellion," but it did become a standpoint through which she interprets the social systems she lives within. In other words, transitioning to natural hair entailed a transition in her consciousness.

Gray used natural hair as a rhetorical tool of resistance. Bringing up stigmas against natural hair in interpersonal interactions redirects attention toward Black women in a conversation about race that often marginalizes their experiences. Gray's body was a political "argumentative resource,"[2] "text,"[3] or symbol to convey her political critique. Against dominant discourses about anti-Black racism in the United States that have largely excluded Black women, Gray, a Black woman without celebrity status, deployed her natural hair to make her personal experience of racism intelligible to others. Natural hair enabled her to connect the daily racist and patriarchal microaggressions she and many other Black women encounter with more privileged narratives, such as the controversy around the Black activist aesthetic of Beyoncé's Super Bowl performance of her song "Formation,"[4] or the widespread media coverage following the murder of Michael Brown in Ferguson, Missouri, which became one of the foremost examples of police brutality in the Black Lives Matter movement.[5] While those with gender or class privilege tend to get more airtime to share and discuss their grievances, many Black women's experiences at the intersection of race, class, and gender oppression are left out of the picture. Single focus discourses about Black men's experiences of racism or celebrity women's experiences of marginalization further challenge Black women's ability to legibly address the complex social problems they face daily as people in simultaneously non-white and non-male bodies, especially in the wake of the new natural hair trend. As Gray explicitly intuited and articulated to Clinton, her beauty and her body had something to say about status quo politics in a particularly tense social moment.

In this chapter, I consider the following question: How does the body, and particularly natural hair, become a vehicle and agent of intersectional resistance? Often, when beauty scholars discuss politics, they often use the term to acknowledge that systems and ideologies of stratification reflect which bodies get what and why. Less understood is how women experience, engage, and critique social movements through beauty culture. And, even though the human body is taken up in *all* social protests, social movement scholarship rarely engages literature on embodiment. Since new collective identities, or shared senses of purpose, are constituted through the gendered, sexed, and racialized body, studying the function of the active and visible body is critical to understanding the goals, strategies, and effects of social movements.[6] That Black women insist on calling natural hair a "movement" rather than a trend is meaningful and telling. So here, I take seriously their claims that natural hair *is* a movement. I begin by situating natural hair politics within Black women's long histories, strategies, and experiences of intersectional activism.

Activism and Intersectionality

Black women activists have long used their situated lived experiences—their standpoints at the intersection of race, class, and gender oppression—to critique priorities of and illuminate gaps within broader anti-racist and feminist conversations. For an early example, formerly enslaved abolitionists and feminists Frederick Douglass and Sojourner Truth were divided on who should receive the right to vote first in mid-nineteenth-century America: women or Black men. Believing that it was the "Negro's hour," at a meeting of the Equal Rights Association on May 14, 1868, Douglass argued, "The government in this country loves women. They are the sisters, mothers, wives and daughters of our rulers; but the negro is loathed . . . The negro needs suffrage to protect his life and property, and to answer him with respect and education."[7] His argument assumed a white female subject, and failed to acknowledge that Black women were rarely embraced as wives and daughters of white leaders but were more often exploited as their property. Black women also experienced exploitation in ways different from their Black male counterparts. For example, the Tignon Laws mandating that Black women cover their hair was a response to the reality that enslaved Black women were more likely to experience sexual violence than enslaved Black men. Sojourner Truth criticized Douglass's position, pointing out Black women's subordinate position to Black men *within* Black communities as well. Perhaps because Truth was also intimately familiar with the experience of patriarchal control, a privilege that Black *and* white men exercise over Black women, she prioritized women's suffrage to protect Black women. Truth claimed, "[Black men] have been having our right so long, that you think, like a slaveholder, that you own us. I know that it is hard for one who has held the reigns for so long to give up; it cuts like a knife. It will feel all better when it closes up again."[8]

Women of color have often faced the pressure to choose allegiance with either men of their same race or with white-centered feminism. Scholars have described this variously as a love vs. trouble[9] or gender vs. race[10] dilemma. Choosing race-centered activism, women of color in the Chicano movement, the African American Civil Rights Movement, and the Black Liberation Movement consistently reported that men minimized their labor, subjectivities, and claims to dignity.[11] As Lorde notes, "The necessity for an history of shared battle have made us, Black women, particularly vulnerable to the false accusation that anti-sexist is anti-Black. Meanwhile, woman-hating as a recourse of the powerless is sapping strength from Black communities and our very lives."[12] Many anti-racist movements, especially ones that employ nationalist frameworks, tend to rest on patriarchal and heteronormative racial uplift strategies that disempower or exclude women of color. For example, in discussing her work with the Black Panther Party at the International

Decolonial Black Feminism Summer School in 2017, scholar-activist Angela Davis mentioned Stokely Carmichael's comment that "the only position for women in [the Student Nonviolent Coordinating Committee] is prone" and recalled when leaders of the Black Panther party put all—and only—the women party members on probation and made them prove their loyalty to the group.[13] Eventually, leaders of the Black Panther Party mandated that members align themselves with only one political group. (Davis chose the Communist Party partly because of her experience with sexism in the Black Panther Party). Gendered double standards extended to the body, as well. Some men in Black Nationalist communities saw natural hair as political for Black men but masculinizing for Black women, a heteronormative stance that suggested that a Black woman's primary role within the movement was as a sexual object for heterosexual Black men.[14] Black lesbians were considered especially threatening to Black Nationalism's pursuit of racial solidarity because they eluded patriarchal control altogether.[15] Meanwhile, others measured women's "consciousness" and commitment to the movement based on their choice and ability to go natural. All in all, as Kristin Denise Rowe documents, Black women were left feeling "policed" and surveilled" by those who should have been their comrades.[16]

Black and Chicana feminists were also routinely ostracized by race and class biases in the second-wave feminism of the 1960s and 1970s.[17] Women of color felt alienated by liberal feminism's conceptualization of a public/private divide, since minority and working-class women have been discriminated against alongside men in their communities and have long worked outside the home to support their families.[18] Feminist organizing on the basis of a monolithic category "woman" ignores that white women have historically and systematically benefitted from white supremacy, and Black feminists in the second wave found that many white feminists had little concern for the issues poor and minority women face.[19] As anti-racist scholar Peggy McIntosh observes, privilege is, by nature, weightless and reproductive, and as a result, is easily invisible to those who benefit from it.[20]

Since feminist and anti-racist movements tend not to acknowledge women of color's experiences of marginalization, feminist organizing along racial/ethnic lines blossomed in the 1960s and 1970s.[21] Through organizations like Hijas de Cuauhtémoc, Organization of Pan Asian American Women, Comisión Femenil Mexicana Nacional, the Combahee River Collective, and the National Black Feminist Organization, women of color pointed out that race and gender justice causes need not be oppositional, since patriarchy upholds racial oppression.[22] Women of color feminists tended to distance themselves from "radical" feminist arguments that advanced separatism to subvert patriarchy, recognizing their common stake with men of color in dismantling racism. For example, writer Alice Walker defines womanism, her version of Black feminism, as "committed to the survival and wholeness of entire people, male *and* female."[23] Black lesbian feminists further argued that aggression against lesbians of color is misplaced, given that the dominant source of violence against Black communities comes from above in existing racist and capitalist social hierarchies.[24] Most famously, the 1977 Combahee River Collective's "Black Feminist Statement" aims to ideologically articulate Black feminism by using their resources as "tokens" within the educational system. The Collective's statement critiques Marxist theory as only partially explanatory of economic oppression, arguing that a socialist revolution can only liberate Black women if it is also anti-racist and feminist. The Collective further describes systems of racist, patriarchal, and capitalist oppression as "interlocking" and mutually-constitutive. Importantly, they posit that their identities as women of color produce particular experiences of racial-sexual oppression, locating the genesis of their anti-racist, anti-sexist, anti-capitalist, and anti-heterosexist politics in their lived struggles for survival.[25]

Academic explanations of the relationships between racism, capitalism, patriarchy, and heteronormativity gained traction in the 1970s and 1980s, perhaps because more women of color were receiving university training and at higher levels than ever before. Scholars of color increasingly interpreted their experiences through theory-making.[26] Women of color feminism made headway in academia through sociologist Patricia Hill Collins's theory of "the matrix of domination," which posits that systems of oppression are interlocking, not simply additive.[27] Similarly, using difference as an analytical lens, critical race scholar Kimberlé Crenshaw introduced the concept of "intersectionality" to describe differential patterns of violence and employment discrimination against women of color. Crenshaw further argued that Black women's experiences of rape and battering become invisible to policymakers, theorists, and activists because of their tendency to see race and gender as mutually-exclusive categories.[28] In turn, laws that conceptualize discrimination along only one axis—either race or gender—frequently dismiss women of color's grievances at the intersection of multiple axes of oppression. The conceptual term "intersectionality," its framework, and the resultant field of study builds upon the knowledge projects of decades of Black activism.[29] Women of color academics increasingly use intersectional frameworks to revise, extend, and critique Eurocentric and androcentric biases across the humanities and social sciences.

Given the birthplaces and historical origins of intersectional thinking—in the social movement communities of women of color—academic intersectionality should always remain in conversation with the forms, foci, and evolutions of Black women's organizing. The natural hair movement is a useful site for documenting the sorts of intersectional knowledge-making Black women find imperative today, especially since concurrent anti-racist social movements often still fail to account for Black women's gendered experiences of racism in their frameworks and discourses. Activism within and through today's natural hair movement is a continuation of Black women's longstanding efforts toward intersectional visibility. Natural hair functions as an ongoing project of embodied intersectional critical praxis that Black women use in response to current political affairs and androcentric frameworks in local political conversations. This is best demonstrated by a cross-cultural comparison of two social movements occurring simultaneously on opposite sides of the Atlantic: Black Lives Matter and the Fees Must Fall protests.

Black Lives Matter and Natural Hair Politics in the United States

In February 2012, Trayvon Martin, a seventeen-year-old Black boy, was murdered by a white Hispanic man named George Zimmerman, who assumed that Martin was causing trouble in his South Florida neighborhood. Zimmerman was acquitted on rationale of self-defense in 2013. The injustice of Martin's death, in addition to many prior and subsequent killings of unarmed Black people by white police and vigilantes, inspired Black queer women activists Alicia Garza, Patrisse Cullors, and Ayọ (formerly known as Opal) Tometi to call for change using the hashtag #BlackLivesMatter on social media. The hashtag and slogan caught on as Black communities aimed to intervene and call attention to the systematic dehumanization, under-recognition, and deadly oppression of Black people and Black bodies. By 2016, the hashtag #BlackLivesMatter had evolved into Black Lives Matter, a decentralized movement and coalition of organizations with over forty chapters across the United States and Canada. The deaths of Trayvon Martin, Michael Brown, Tamir Rice, Eric Garner, and many, many others woke up the nation to a much too common form of tragedy. By 2020, due in large part to outrage at the murder of George Floyd in Minneapolis by police officer Derek Chauvin, Black Lives Matter had become one of the largest social movements in US history.

Say Her Name: Gendering Black Lives Matter

As the movement and initiative grew, the dominant narrative advanced by grassroots activists and media portrayals seemed to center police brutality against cisgender men to the exclusion of women and trans people. Although Garza, Cullors, and Tometi publicly and repeatedly used their platforms to advance gendered analyses of state and white supremacist violence, violence against Black cis and trans women have not inspired the same level of outrage that violence against Black cis men's bodies has. The tragedies of Black women like Sandra Bland, Rekia Boyd, Tanisha

Anderson, Yvette Smith, and many others who have been assaulted, killed, or violently intimidated by the police have rallied less attention. Crenshaw et al. lament this situation: "The erasure of Black women is not purely a matter of missing facts. Even where women and girls are present in the data, narratives framing police profiling and lethal force as exclusively male experiences lead researchers, the media, and advocates to exclude them."[30] Now, as in the past, Black women are not commonly viewed as representative recipients of the violence of white supremacy.

In May 2015, the #SayHerName social media initiative was a major public step toward recognizing and remembering Black American women's experiences of police violence. Brown et al. analyze #SayHerName as a case study of intersectional critical practice and consciousness-raising in the digital era, whereby racism and sexism are simultaneously interrogated through social media networks to center trans and cis Black women's deaths.[31] While #SayHerName has importantly raised awareness that not "all the Blacks are men," the campaign has done little to describe and illustrate the gendered ways in which Black women encounter racism.[32] Beginning with a narrative of police brutality occurring on the street eclipses other, more common ways in which Black women experience violence and racism. In an interview with Kaavya Asoka for the academic journal *Dissent*, scholar Marcia Chatelain suggests the greater likelihood for Black women to experience violence in the private sphere as an explanation for their erasure from Black Lives Matter discourses about anti-Black violence. Chatelain offers:

> Black women are often targets of violence inside homes and in private spaces where people cannot easily see them or galvanize around them. When we consider how and where people organize, it's important to remember these victims of brutality too, even if we can't gather at their specific sites of victimization.[33]

In other words, violence against Black women often looks different from violence against Black men, often taking the forms of sexual harassment, rape, and other unwanted touching. Amid a men-centered, street-centered movement against racial violence, the natural hair movement has become a way for Black women to make their lived experiences of racism and their right to bodily integrity visible and legible.

Don't Touch My Hair: Black Women and Bodily Integrity

In November 2017, I heard model and activist Ebonee Davis speak on a panel titled "Race and Fashion," where she described how her standpoint as a woman with natural hair and one of few Black models in high fashion revealed to her the role of racist and limited media representations in perpetuating violence and implicit biases against Black bodies. She described how, early in her career, modeling agencies repeatedly declined to represent her because their company portfolios already had their token Black models. Those that did agree to sign her used her as their "backup Black girl" when their other Black models were unavailable. It was not until Davis became a spokesperson for diversity issues through a viral 2017 TED Talk on "Black Girl Magic in the Fashion Industry" that an agency seeking models who could work in the influencer branding space agreed to represent her. Davis opened her TED Talk with an anecdote from her childhood, where she remembers begging her grandmother for a box of relaxer at the beauty supply store so that she could have beautiful straight hair and abandon her "kinky coils." She spoke of makeup artists painting her gray, too careless to properly match her shade, and stylists' inability to work with her hair, forcing her to big chop.[34] On the day Davis went natural in July 2016, Alton Sterling was shot and killed by police officers in Louisiana.[35] The coincidence inspired a critical reflection on the relationships between racism, fashion, and violence. In her public letter for *Harper's Bazaar*, Davis uses analogies to beauty and hair as an argumentative resource:

> It is the same systemic racism that sees beauty products for "Black" hair
> end up in a section of their own ("the ethnic aisle"), that sees Black men

more likely to end up dead after a police encounter than any other racial group. Systemic racism began with slavery and has woven itself into the fabric of our culture, manifesting through police brutality, poverty, lack of education, and incarceration. The most dangerous contributors? Advertising, beauty, and fashion.[36]

Davis's letter demands that the beauty industry expand the definition of beauty to be racially inclusive, rather than forcing Black, Latina, Arab, and Asian women to assimilate into white-centered beauty norms: "We have a responsibility to re-humanize the systematically dehumanized, and create of a society where each of us can be recognized, represented, and celebrated across the board, so we can take pride in who we are and where we come from."[37] Here, Davis uses natural hair and beauty as rhetorical tools for connecting Black women's experiences negotiating a white-centered beauty ideal and beauty industry with the movement to end police brutality. Davis's experience also highlights the distinctive and powerful role of social media "influencers" as political spokespersons in today's digital era.

I observed several other convergences between discourses in the natural hair movement and the Black Lives Matter movement. The public conversation around police officers' implicit bias against Black men in hoodies mirrored an ongoing conversation about employers' implicit bias against natural hair in schools, in transit, and in workplaces. Legal cases regulating hair discrimination have been widely publicized since the 1980s, like *Rogers v. American Airlines* in 1981 and a 2016 Eleventh Circuit Federal Court of Appeals decision that protects employers who fire employees with locs.[38] The Perception Institute's 2017 "'Good Hair' Study" received extensive media attention for comparing implicit bias against Black women wearing natural versus straightened hair styles. The study found that most participants in its national sample of Black and white men and women, regardless of race, show implicit bias against Black women with natural hair textures.[39]

As I hopped from one natural hair event to another during my field-work, I was surprised to discover that one of the most common topics discussed not directly connected to beauty care was state violence and the criminalization of Black girls. One particular natural hair event I attended in 2016 in Los Angeles stands out in my field notes, during which the organizer connected hair relaxing to reproductive injustice, mass incarceration, and domestic violence. She distributed a handout that informed attendees that there had been an 832% increase in the incarceration of women of color in the United States since 1977, cor-related by increased prison privatization. While a conversation about prison privatization as a racial justice issue had gaining attention at the time thanks to legal scholar Michelle Alexander's now-iconic text *The New Jim Crow* (2010), such analyses have focused primarily on incarcer-ated Black men and, indirectly, the women who love and care for them. However, the leader of this natural hair event emphasized the unique and direct effects incarceration has on Black women, explaining how incarcerated women are forced to give birth in shackles. Yet, she pointed out, there is no data tying health records to prison records. Describ-ing both relaxers and maternal healthcare in the prison system as forms of gender-based violence that alienate women from their own bodies, she continued, "Knowing this data helps to embrace our sisters and to understand Black beauty politics. The women I work with can't trust their bodies to do anything. We need to know more and go deeper. It is our responsibility to find out more." African American women's discus-sions connecting the Black beauty politics with police violence and the prison industrial complex do not occur in a vacuum. They draw upon the history of the surveillance and criminalization of Black women's bodies. Specifically, they speak to enduring cultural associations of the Afro-wearing Black woman with violent Black radicalism. Recall that hundreds or thousands of Afro-wearing Black women were harassed by the police when Angela Davis's image was circulated by the FBI in 1970. One protestor, seen during fieldwork at a Black Lives Matter protest in

FIGURE 4.1. Protester at a Black
Lives Matter rally. Author's photo.

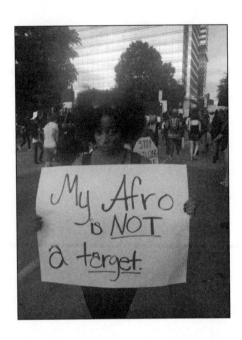

Atlanta, Georgia, evokes this history in her sign that read "My Afro is
NOT a TARGET."

A focus on bodily integrity and personal safety among natural hair
communities in the United States also responds to Black Lives Matter's
anti-violence emphasis. In talking about their experiences of gendered
racism, numerous women I interviewed and met in the field referenced
instances where they warded off invasive touches and disparaging comments from friends and strangers. Such instances are reminders of and
speak to a long history of treating Black women like spectacles and
raiding their personal space. "Don't touch my hair" has become central slogan of the natural hair movement, appearing repeatedly in recent music, books, natural hair forums, and newspaper articles. As of
December 2021, there are over 114k images tagged #donttouchmyhair
on Instagram, mostly "selfies" or self-portraits of Black women with
natural hair. In 2016, comedian Phoebe Robinson published her best-
selling book on race, gender, and pop culture titled *You Can't Touch My*

Hair—part media analysis, part memoir of the various racist and sexist microaggressions she faced growing up and working in the entertainment industry. Also in 2016, Solange Knowles released her song "Don't Touch My Hair." Knowles's song is in many ways the contemporary response to India Arie's 2006 hit single "I Am Not My Hair," released exactly ten years earlier. While Arie emphasizes that her soul is "within," Knowles posits that her hair *is* her soul, her pride, her emotions—and is off limits. In a recorded conversation with her mother for her website Saint Heron, Knowles explicitly connects her album to the movement against police brutality:

> When I felt afraid or when I felt like this record would be so different from my last, I would see or hear another story of a young Black person in America having their life taken away and having their freedom taken away. That would fuel me to go back and revisit and sometimes rewrite some of these songs to go a little further and not be afraid to have the conversation.[40]

Knowles's music video for "Don't Touch My Hair" features her and other feminine Black women and men in a rotating array of hairstyles, including beaded cornrows with cowrie shells, finger waves, and curly 'fros. The aesthetic is distinctly Black, but necessarily Afrocentric. It projects Black hair as playful, creative, and personal. Unlike the 1970s Black Power slogan "Black Is Beautiful" that focused on rearticulating and celebrating an Afrocentrist aesthetic, the 2010s slogan "Don't Touch My Hair" is a directive to others and a demand for bodily respect.

In 2013, Antonia Opiah of natural hair website Un-ruly challenged the "Don't Touch My Hair" idea through a social experiment entitled "You Can Touch My Hair." For the experiment, three volunteers held signs inviting strangers in Union Square, New York, to feel their hair without consequence. Opiah intended to inspire cultural exchange and undercut the curiosity around Black hair. In a blog post for the *Huffington Post* she explained, "Hair was the vulnerability that we offered up, a bargaining chip we hoped would get us what we really want—one brick on the bridge we need to really integrate as Americans."[41] Unsurprisingly, the experiment sparked a voracious debate on social media and in real life. Some welcomed the conversation it began, which gave Black women another platform to explain the significance of the natural hair movement and the daily microaggressions they face because of their hair. Others likened the experiment to a slave auction block, a petting zoo, and the infamous exhibition of Sarah Baartman's naked body for white enjoyment around Europe in the early 1800s.[42] On the second day of Opiah's experiment, a group of women staged counterprotests, carrying signs saying "What'll it be next . . . my butt?" and "Don't know where your hands have been, so no."

The counterprotesters pointed out that curiosity cannot be benign in a society defined by white supremacy and against the backdrop of centuries of racist and sexist violence against Black women's bodies. Similarly, sociologist George Yancey powerfully explains:

> Whether the white hand touches in the form of gentle embrace or touches out of curiosity, what is important is that the Black woman expresses deep discomfort; she is not pleased, and she clearly does not want or desire to be touched. After all, the history of whiteness demonstrates that curious white hands can lead to violent acts of objectifying and experimenting on Black bodies; and desirous white hands can lead to violent and unspeakable acts of molestation, where the Black body undergoes tremendous pain and trauma.[43]

The refrain "Don't Touch My Hair" encapsulates this reality, demanding changes in the treatment of Black women. These critiques of invasive microaggressions against natural hair do important work in highlighting patriarchal forms of violence against Black women's bodies in the United States alongside Black Lives Matter.

Fees Must Fall and Natural Hair Politics in South Africa

Like all racial formation projects, today's natural hair movement in South Africa is shaped by the country's history and engages current political affairs. Apartheid ended with South Africa's democratic election in 1994, when the African National Congress (ANC) won and elected Nelson Mandela president. Archbishop Desmond Tutu predicted that democratic South Africa would become the "rainbow nation"—a place where a diverse and multicultural population would live in peaceful coexistence.[44] However, upon Mandela's death in 2013, the country was forced to reflect on the ANC's promise and vision of a multicultural, harmonic, and unified society. The ANC's stated vision of a "South Africa that belongs to all who live in it, Black and white" had not manifested twenty years after the end of apartheid.[45] South African society and particularly Black and Coloured South Africans were reconsidering and reevaluating the rainbow nation ideal with disappointment. The ANC's central defining commitment to non-racialism was even receiving critique from within the party for enabling white supremacist institutional and cultural racism to thrive.[46] Then in August 2016, the ANC faced its worst election loss post-apartheid.

The radical leftist Economic Freedom Fighter (EFF) party, led by Julius Malema, came in a distant third in the 2016 election, but the party's heightened visibility symbolized a growing demand for racialized pathways to social justice. Malema drew support with promises to redistribute land still controlled by wealthy whites to poor Black South Africans—a solution that the ANC and Democratic Alliance (DA) have shied away from. Malema's Black Nationalist and socialist vision for South Africa, including free education through college, appealed to younger voters. While many millennial and older South Africans of color believe in the potential of assimilating into a multiracial South African elite, the so-called "born free" and newly-enfranchised generation is more skeptical.[47] Over twenty years into democracy, race and racism continue to structure South Africa's educational system, geography, economic system, and political power elite.

The Fees Must Fall and Rhodes Must Fall student movements arose from young South Africans' growing discontent with persistent inequality and the ANC's failure to redistribute land, space, and resources to South Africa's people of color. In March 2016, a group of students at the University of Cape Town (UCT) protested for the removal of a statue of imperialist and miner Cecil Rhodes, an infamous force for British settler colonialism in South Africa.[48] Since 1934, the larger-than-life figure has perched high on Table Mountain, literally gazing down upon the Cape Flats, an economically impoverished and predominantly Coloured township. Rhodes Must Fall protestors argued that the statue emblematized racial and colonial oppression, a physical representation of how white supremacy continues to spatially, ideologically, and demographically shape UCT. Activists' arguments echo Steve Biko's Black Consciousness critique of integration forty years earlier, which cautioned against South African Blacks "assimilating into an already established set of norms and code of behavior set up by and maintained by whites."[49] By the time the August 2016 elections rolled around, Rhodes Must Fall had garnered the support of tens of thousands of students at universities across South Africa including North-West University, University of the Free State, University of Witwatersand, University of Pretoria, and the University of KwaZulu-Natal, and later in the UK at Oxford University where a similar statue stands. (The statue of Cecil Rhodes was eventually taken down at UCT, but a similar one survived at Oxford.) The growing outrage was more than symbolic or ideological. Black and Coloured South African students are underrepresented at UCT despite their demographic majority not just in the Cape Town metropolitan area, but also nationwide.

The Rhodes Must Fall initiative evolved into the nationwide Fees Must Fall student movement, taking on an anti-capitalist orientation in September 2016, when the South African Minister of Higher Education announced plans to increase tuition at all universities. Fees Must Fall became the largest student revolt since the anti-apartheid Soweto uprising of 1976.[50] Deploying a broad understanding of Blackness that included other poor, rural, and socially marginalized non-whites, the Fees Must Fall movement called for free, decolonized education for all. Youth across the country took to the streets, burning down centuries-old paintings of colonizers and setting libraries ablaze. Fees Must Fall and Rhodes Must Fall student activists occupied an administrative building at UCT, renaming it Azania House,[51] and transformed it into a space "removed from the white gaze and also from the violent constructions of Blackness in which other University spaces inform."[52] After students set fire to centuries-old artwork and literature from the colonial era, several universities hired private security firms to protect their assets; their guards shot protestors with rubber bullets and surveilled and patrolled campuses through the night. When I went to meet students at the university, I was greeted by dozens of marching young people who went from building to building in the rain, marching, singing, and recruiting additional protesters from classrooms. UCT, University of Witwatersrand, and University of KwaZulu-Natal ultimately canceled final exams, and there was a general sense of anxiety about how Fees Must Fall would affect the national job market. This racial and economic discontent, prominently targeting the educational system, was the immediate context surrounding my ethnographic fieldwork about South Africa's natural hair movement, which took place from August to November 2016.

Fees Must Fall and Feminism

"The similarity between Fees Must Fall and Black Lives Matter is that women were at the forefront of those movements and there was a lot of centering of men, because men are seen as revolutionary."
—Julie (26, Cape Town)

I met Julie, a former UCT law student, through mutual friends engaged in feminist organizing in Cape Town. Due to her involvement in the

Rhodes Must Fall and Fees Must Fall movements and the burning of university artwork, Julie was expelled from UCT and banned from setting foot on campus. Born to an activist family who lived in exile in Europe during her childhood and still runs feminist consciousness raising groups with Black and Coloured farmworkers, Julie's approach to Fees and Rhodes Must Fall was strategic, determined, and unyielding. Her intimate involvement with and eventual separation from campus politics fostered insightful perspective and reflection about the gender and sexual dynamics of the movements, which she hoped would advance a radical Black feminist agenda. As part of her ongoing work, Julie and her comrades organized house parties where admission fees went toward university tuition for UCT's queer and trans population. Julie explained, "One of the ideological pillars was Black radical feminism, and through that, intersectionality. There was a critical way of looking at gender in the movement, through the movement, and through movement exercise." Her political framework stemmed from bell hooks's work critiquing patriarchy and heteronormativity, seeing these systems as inherently intertwined with capitalism and white supremacy.[53] Julie expounded, "In order to achieve liberation, in order to achieve decolonization of our education and society we need to dismantle white supremacy, ableism, capitalism, and patriarchy." However, not all Fees Must Fall organizers agreed with her perspective. Julie faced antagonism from male peers, which threatened to fracture the movement. When I asked how this manifested, Julie explained:

> There was the denial of the privilege of being a man. They'd say, let's deal with race and class now and gender at a later stage. No, fuck that. In previous liberation movements and struggles gender was put on the back burner and now it is time to center it in the work that we're doing.

Rebecca, a 22-year-old African American student studying abroad at the University of Cape Town, who happened to be conducting an ethnography about the gender politics of Fees Must Fall for her under-graduate senior thesis from July to November 2016, likewise observed:

> Something that I noticed was that gender and sexuality were just con-stantly being brought up without explicitly being said. They definitely tried to address rape culture in their pillars and statements but when it came down to actual organizing tactics, their inability to address these issues led to a lot of huge problems. There would be times that we'd be in meetings and issues of hypermasculinity would just dissolve the en-tire meeting. We couldn't even talk anymore, though it needed to get ad-dressed especially as the movement got ramped up and then shut down with the military that [UCT] hired. We tried to define the space. It never really got solved, but it kept coming up. Rifts between the hypermascu-linity of the protestors and the hypermasculinity of the police would just escalate the entire thing.

Movement organizers put on an exhibition called "Trans Capture" to highlight Fees Must Fall's accomplishments. The show attempted to in-clude gender and sexuality as axes of identity and unjust oppression that operate alongside racism and capitalism, but the trans community saw it as disingenuous and tokenizing. Julie's fellow Black radical feminists grew frustrated. "We can't fucking deal," she reflected.

The Fees Must Fall protests that erupted in South Africa's Gauteng province, where Johannesburg and Pretoria are located, suffered similar issues with heteropatriarchy. Based on their survey of one hundred stu-dents at the University of Witwatersrand and the University of Johan-nesburg involved in Fees Must Fall, political scientists Ojakorotu Victor and Esuola Olukayode Segun found that male protestors were motivated not only by the goals of the movement, but also to a great degree by their egotistic desire to protect and possess fellow women students' bod-ies.[54] Victor and Segun analyzed their findings through a heteronorma-tive lens, arguing that women should strive to be complementary rather than competitive with men to achieve political goals because women's mere presence encourages men: "Women, when they participate in politics, often motivate men through their bodies and through psychological factors as men who see themselves as superior will never wait to be counted out when women are in action."[55] This view is incompatible with the radical Black feminist perspective advanced by many women and gender-nonconforming protestors at UCT, who see racism, capitalism, heteronormativity, and patriarchy as interlocking and mutually constitutive. And, as Julie's reflections demonstrate, the experiences of being considered inferior to men and movement leaders' dismissal of non-cismen's concerns are understandably violent and oppressive.

Hair, Hairstyling, and Women of Color's Right to Educational Spaces

Wearing natural hair and public hairstyling protests were often used in by student protesters to express the gendered experience of living and studying in colonized space. Julie recalled a day where women and femme non-binary Fees Must Fall protestors sat in front of Azania House and braided each other's hair with pink and purple fiber (hair used for braiding): "So what if my fiber is blonde, white, purple or whatever. There shouldn't be a stereotypical idea of what your Blackness and femaleness should be. It is that you have the agency to be whatever you want to be and to do that. That was really empowering in that way." When protest is expressed through the body, particularly through feminine displays and cultural forms, it is particularly powerful because it challenges the existing patriarchal order.[56] Women's bodies represented not only a specific form of racial suffering in South Africa, but also intersectional resistance and renewal. Julie described the moment as a form of collective caretaking and Black feminist solidarity that was especially resistant as it occurred in public space, since women's beauty work is often invisible or takes place in the private sphere. Hair braiding at Azania House did not simply challenge the activist narratives around space and belonging in South Africa; it showed that patriarchal heteronormativity affects Black and Coloured women's experiences of racism in ways that differ from men of color. The hair braiding protest challenged both UCT and Fees Must Fall cultures, which similarly compelled women students to adhere to white-centric and patriarchal standards for feminine professionalism and beauty.

Natural hair was also the centerpiece of girls' demands for decolonized education in primary and secondary schools, which garnered international media attention.[57] The same month that UCT students braided each other's hair at Azania House, young high school students at Pretoria Girls High School took to the streets to protest policies requiring them to straighten their hair and banning them from wearing large braids or locs. They carried handmade posters with slogans like "Fists up, 'Fros out," "I was born with nappy hair, deal with it!," and "My hair doesn't need fixing! Society's view of BLACKNESS is what is broken!" Afros were not explicitly mentioned in the school's extensive grooming policy, but students complained that teachers forced them to chemically straighten their hair so as to not appear untidy. Teachers also allegedly told students with locs that their hair looked like bird nests, and students recalled being pulled out of class and given Vaseline to slick down their hair. Black students were also forbidden to speak their native languages at school or hang out in large groups together.

Pretoria Girls High School was founded in 1902 and only allowed white students during apartheid. It admitted its first non-diplomatic student of color in 1991. In many elite, formerly white private schools like Pretoria Girls, grooming rules banning cultural signifiers routinely become obstacles for students of color, particularly feminine students, who are more likely to wear their hair long.[58] Schools surveil and control their bodies through such rules. As Marley, a 26-year-old mathematics teacher in Cape Town explained, "It becomes part of discipline and if your hair isn't *disciplined* to the back you are ill-disciplined." Despite the multiple racially and culturally discriminatory policies girls of color are subjected to at Pretoria Girls High, UCT, and elsewhere, hair became the focal point of young women's protest for their right to take up space in South Africa's elite schools. Sheila, whose daughter attends a neighboring school to Pretoria Girls High School, told me:

> The hair rules there are for us. Nobody else. [White girls'] hair, they never see as funky. I don't understand what that means, but obviously, it is meant for us more than anything. But it happens everywhere— whether it is in semi-model C schools [former whites-only government schools]—but obviously at public schools it often doesn't happen because it is our space so nobody will give a policy that will oppress people who look like you.

Tens of thousands of people signed online petitions to combat racism at Pretoria Girls High by dismantling the grooming policy, and the protest preoccupied political conversation on national media outlets for weeks. The upper echelon of South Africa's political scene all weighed in on Twitter and on television. The Democratic Alliance and the African National Congress Women's League both issued statements in support of the girls.[59] Eventually, the head of education in Gauteng province ordered an independent audit of racism at the school, and the code of conduct was revised.

Focusing on hair advanced an intersectional critique of broader Fees Must Fall narratives that lacked an analysis of belonging. Wearing natural hair at school became a symbolic celebration of Black beauty that aimed to reorganize and redistribute resources along intersecting race, class, and gender lines. By embracing a racialized physical feature, women and girl students rejected the requirement that they adhere to Eurocentric standards to receive education, be upwardly mobile, and pursue economic security. In other words, the natural hair protests were Black feminist racial formation projects: Black by affirming a Black aesthetic, feminist by centering women, decolonial by subverting colonially-defined spatial boundaries.

Individual Resistance vs. Collective Action: A Generational Gap

While South Africa's "born free" generation uses natural hairstyling primarily in contexts of collective protest, the millennial and Generation X women of color I interviewed continued to be isolated in their professional environments and negotiated hair politics on an individual basis. For these women, conversations about the resistant nature of natural hair usually begin and end online. Many of the older women I interviewed described feeling pressured to straighten their hair to assimilate into newly accessible elite institutions in alignment with the rainbow nation frameworks, which deemphasized racial difference in an effort to move toward equality, that dominated South Africa's understanding of reconciliation and nation-building when they came of age. Zina (27, Johannesburg) felt proud of the Pretoria Girls High students. She told me that she felt insecure about whether the opportunities now available to her as a Black woman would be sacrificed if she transgressed Eurocentric standards of beauty and professionalism, and she felt this risk acutely as the daughter of an anti-apartheid freedom fighter who spent years as a political prisoner on Robben Island, where Nelson Mandela was also imprisoned. Likewise, Sheila observed a reluctance to fight school grooming rules against Afros among her parent peers, explaining, "It's really important that we as parents stand up to this because I've tried doing it with other parents and they distance themselves from me. You're too political. Everything is okay. When you're too political it's going to destabilize things." As a historically specific manifestation of and response to race, class, and gender arrangements, the 2016 natural hair protests (as with Fees Must Fall more broadly) were interpreted differently by different generations, who have had divergent experiences with the state and in society. Both apartheid barriers and rainbow nation ideals live on through social structures, as well as in peoples' hopes, fears, and memories of segregation and exclusion.

Global Culture, Local Politics

A comparison of natural hair discourses in South Africa and the United States shows that natural hair is political, but not necessarily a cohesive movement in and of itself for the people who participate in and feed it. Like the Afro of the 1960s and 1970s, natural hair is a symbol, expressed through bodies, with relative and contextual meanings. State-level conflicts determine the direction of local natural hair communities' political critique: institutional exclusion in South Africa and bodily integrity in the United States, for examples.

Black women's deployment of beauty politics transfers frames developed in other highly-publicized racial justice movements occurring at the same place and time. Meyer and Whittier call this symbiotic transmission of activist symbolism, orientation, and strategy "social movement spillover," and suggest that the transference of social movement frames is greatest when group membership overlaps.[60] While there is much international overlap in the discourse on natural hair care, fashion, and Black-affirming aesthetics, there is less overlap in membership of anti-racist social movements employing on-the-ground protest strategies. So, natural hair is deployed to different ends in local contexts, where participants in natural hair culture are simultaneously members of or sympathizers with the social movement organizations in the communities in which they live. In other words, while natural hair culture is global in scope, its meanings and applications are shaped by local histories, racial regimes, geographies, and social movements.

Even as gendered racial projects and expressions of embodied intersectional praxis are locally and historically situated, in a rapidly globalizing world social movements across the Black Atlantic often find inspiration from and solidarity with one another. Global Black feminist networks and discourses circulate both digitally and physically across the Black Atlantic, spreading Black feminist analyses of gendered racism. Recall that Julie (26, Cape Town) used American scholar bell hooks's theoretical framework as the basis of her politics, comparing the

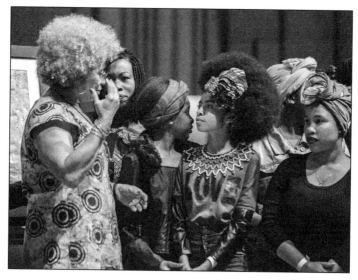

FIGURE 4.2. Angela Davis with Zulaikha Patel, a student at Pretoria Girls High School, Dougan, Laila Lee. 2016. "Policing black women's hair." *Africasacountry.com.*

marginalization of women and trans people within the Fees Must Fall movement to androcentric orientations in Black Lives Matter. Diasporic groups use one another as resources, especially if they are struggling against similar postcolonial, capitalist, white supremacist, and patriarchal structures. In addition, the Pretoria Girls hair protests garnered international attention by the likes of the *New York Times, Washington Post, BBC,* and the *Guardian,* among many others, spurring transnational social media conversations about implicit bias against natural hair in the workplace and in schools.[61] The hashtag #StopRacismAtPretoriaGirlsHigh was used over 150,000 times on Twitter. Angela Davis discussed links between the criminalization of her Afro in the 1970s and hair rules at a talk at Pretoria Girls High with Zulaikha Patel, who became the unofficial spokesperson for the Pretoria Girls hair protests. Six months later, Angela Davis and I compared our sentiments about the Pretoria Girls protests at the International Decolonial Black Feminism Summer School in Cachoeira, Brazil. These exchanges evidence the global, networked nature of Black feminism. Political thought, including decolonial Black feminist thought, transcends state boundaries. These examples highlight how racial formation projects can be simultaneously global, local, interpersonal, and embodied.

Conclusion

In an effort to make their particular experiences of racism visible and legible, Black and Coloured women are using natural hair as an intersectional political tool to connect gendered forms of racism with more dominant, androcentric conversations occurring among communities engaged in political change in a given place and time. In other words, natural hair has become embodied intersectional critical praxis—a tool for critiquing dominant social and political discourses that elevate one category of analysis above others, such as men's experiences of white supremacist racism.[62] Women in both South Africa and in the United States use natural hair as an embodied intersectional interjection into broad conversations about politics, where dominant discourses often erase their experiences by centering men's bodily integrity (in the United States) and right to take up space (in South Africa).

A comparison of natural hair protests in South Africa and the United States shows how the ways in which women apply natural hair as an argumentative resource responds to political debates in overlapping local social movement circles. The differences in how South African and US women use natural hair in their critiques highlights how "different social movement cultures, specific movement demands, and activists' differential locations in the social structure shape embodied actions" and their meanings.[63] And so, while natural hair culture transgresses national boundaries and has united women across the African diaspora, what it means to be natural depends upon the local conflicts, contexts, and histories in which they live.

5

Who Can Be Natural?

Privilege and Exclusion

"Subversion is contextual, historical, and above all social.
No matter how exciting the 'destabilizing' potential of texts,
bodily or otherwise, whether texts are subversive or recuper-
ative or both or neither cannot be determined by abstraction
from actual social practice."
—Susan Bordo, *Unbearable Weight: Feminism, Western
Culture, and the Body*

In June 2015, Rachel Dolezal catapulted from relative obscurity in the
small city of Spokane, Washington, to worldwide fame when her local
television station, with the help of her biological parents who both identify as Caucasian, exposed that she'd been passing as Black for years.
Much of the fascination around Dolezal centered around her embodied
performance of race. Formerly blonde-haired and blue-eyed, over the
course of a decade Dolezal physically transformed her appearance using
spray tans and skillfully installed curly wigs, kinky weaves, faux locs, and
micro braids. On her birthday in 2013, two years before her story became
a global sensation, she posted a trio of mirror selfies that later went viral
of herself with sandy brown spiral curls and the caption, "Going with the
natural look as I start my 36th year."[1] Since hair texture is a key signifier
of Blackness, her embrace of braids and curly "natural" weaves helped
her accomplish a Black identity that her community accepted.[2] At the
time, Dolezal was president of Spokane's NAACP chapter and an adjunct
professor in Africana Studies at nearby Eastern Washington University.
Natural hair seemed to embody her anti-racist political and academic

work. Dolezal was well-read on the politics and history of Black hair; video clips of her PowerPoint lectures on such topics surfaced online in the wake of the media saga that ensued through the summer of 2015. In fact, over a decade earlier, she had written and illustrated a book called *Ebony Tresses* for her Black adopted sister that celebrated the power in her sister's kinky hair.[3] In the aftermath of the media controversy and as she struggled to find work, Dolezal began making a living braiding hair and installing weaves for Black women in her community. Kara Brown wrote for *Jezebel*, "clearly Rachel knew: Those spray tans would not be enough. The hair—she had to nail the hair—and boy did she."[4] Against the legacy of the "one-drop rule" of hypodescent in the United States, which legally categorized persons with any degree of African ancestry as Black regardless of phenotype, ethnicity, or migration history, it seemed that few who knew Dolezal questioned her claim to a Black racial identity because of her light skin. Her lightness did not prevent her from participating in Blackness, but it did enable her to capitalize on colorism and white privilege.

Regardless of Dolezal's long record of public, private, and embodied resistances to white supremacist racism, many were offended by her claim to a Black racial identity, criticizing her for culturally appropriating Black hairstyles and arguing that she could never understand the lived experience of Black womanhood. Much of this criticism circulated online, making #AskRachel one of Black Twitter's most popular hashtags in 2015. Through #AskRachel, people created a series of ironic memes that presumed common experiences of Blackness, implying that those who couldn't answer weren't truly Black or Black enough: For example, is a kitchen a room where you cook food or the fluff of tight coils at the nape of someone's neck? If you can't answer, the meme implies, you can't claim Blackness. By questioning Dolezal's racial authenticity, her critics further questioned her right to engage in identity politics and Black cultural forms, particularly through the body. Political scientist Joseph Lowndes used the term "political blackface" to accuse Dolezal of stealing Black intellectual and political leadership.[5] The criticism of and conflict around Dolezal increased doubt about hair texture and skin color as tools for assessing, accomplishing, or inhabiting Blackness and highlight a perspective that racial authenticity should be a requisite for engaging in identity politics. As a result, several multiracial bloggers blamed Dolezal for increased and invasive demands that they also "prove their Blackness" through narrating experiences of racial discrimination and performing cultural knowledge. That's why I find the Dolezal controversy compelling—it embodies dynamics I observed in the natural hair movement. Similar debates about whether "natural" hairstyles are meaningful and acceptable for white, multi-racial, and light-skinned women probe the fragile boundary around the natural hair movement's collective political identity. As the quote by Susan Bordo at the opening of this chapter asserts, the resistant and political meanings and effects of an act—like participating in natural hair culture—cannot be divorced from the relational contexts between fellow doers and observers. Racial histories, texture hierarchies, and capitalist pressures complicate who can exist comfortably in the natural hair movement. Given that, this chapter unpacks a set of very basic, yet fundamentally important, questions: *Who can be natural, where, and why?*

Forming a Collective Identity around Natural Hair

To understand *who can be natural,* one first needs to understand how critical of a role identity has come to play in the twenty-first-century political landscape. I place natural hair politics within the scholarly conversation on new social movements, which are characterized by their concern with cultural validation, individual autonomy, and self-transformation, as opposed to traditional social movements that focus on class arrangements, operate through formal organizations, and appeal for state change.[6] Observing trends in feminist, LGBTQ, and green movements, scholars argue that new social movements are characterized by their strategic politicization of collective identity to portray claims to political power, material resources, and representational control.[7] Born out of the study of new social movements, collective identity theory focuses on how groups construct and negotiate boundaries to create insiders who share common grievances and political outlooks, as well as outsiders, who are seen as oppressors.[8] In other words, "boundary markers . . . frame the interaction between members of the in-group and the out-group."[9] Taylor and Whittier further argue that "collective political actors do not exist *de facto* by virtue of individuals sharing a common structural location," but that collective identities are strategically invoked to demarcate oppositional boundaries between the oppressed group and others.[10] Correspondingly, collective identity theory understands all identities, including racial and gender identities, as socially constructed projects. To understand how new social movements participate in race and gender evolution, we must examine how and whether groups invoke, reconstruct, or de-emphasize race and gender in appeals for material, political, and representational power.[11]

For decades, Black feminists have politicized identity to form intellectual, social, and activist communities that reflect how racism, capitalism, and patriarchy mutually shape their lived experiences in unique ways.[12] The collective identity approach challenges us to not take the category "Black woman" as static, cohesive, or for granted. Instead, it encourages scholars to unpack how groups come to draw boundaries around Black womanhood to advance their political agendas. In a rare example that centers the experiences of women of color, scholar-activist Julia Chinyere Oparah[13] uses collective identity theory to frame how African, Asian, and Caribbean women in Great Britain struggle to construct an effective multiracial "Black" collective identity to advance shared political concerns like immigration policy and reproductive rights. Chinyere Oparah finds that Black British women's movement groups emphasize postcolonial history in boundary-making, and must de-emphasize differences in immigration history, nationality, age, location, and ethnic stereotypes to form successful multiracial alliances.[14]

Following a similar analytical lens and approach, this chapter uses interview and ethnographic data alongside media analyses to discuss how women who participate in natural hair politics delimit the group for which the natural hair movement is mean to advocate. In what follows, I describe both Black women's boundary-making and the forces they confront, critique, and organize against. As I will show, most women in the natural hair movement tend to view centering Blackness as a strategy for resisting prevailing white-centered beauty ideals, Black people's displacement from the ethnic haircare market, and limited representations of Black women in the media. Theorizing Black women's activist strategies in the twenty-first century, Brittney Cooper asserts that "our commitment to discursive acts must be measured—by our histories, by our material realities, by the psychic and social costs, and by the attendant benefits of such acts for improving the quality of [our lives]."[15] In other words, the women who participate in natural hair politics actively position and police boundaries around natural hair culture in ways unavoidably constrained and informed by race, class, and gender power relations. Their resultant cultural and material realities—from controlling images of Black women rooted in dominant ideologies to discrimination in the workplace—have often taken up kinky hair as symbolic of Black women's inferiority.[16] The investment in drawing racial boundaries around the natural hair movement's collective identity is also rooted in a four-hundred-years-long battle for power over Black hair's political symbolism, as well as the twentieth-century economics of the Black beauty market. That makes natural hair politics a fruitful opportunity to center intersectionality, the body, and the political economy in collective identity theory—a critically important move in a moment where individualism, autonomy, self-fashioning, and choice challenge previously taken-for-granted categories, but also produce new anxieties about exploitative and opportunistic identity claims.[17]

Policing Access, Authenticity, and Appropriation

Most often, natural hair communities invoke racial boundaries by accusing individuals of cultural appropriation—a topic that flourished in online spaces in the 2010s. Cultural appropriation refers to when "members of one culture [take] something that originates in another cultural context."[18] While most academic researchers discuss cultural appropriation in a value-free sense, natural hair communities and Black internet communities more broadly use the term to imply an exploitative and fetishistic adoption of hairstyles originating from Africa or the African diaspora by non-Black women. In online and in-person conversations, I observed as women in natural hair communities expressed disdain for white women who wear braids, cornrows, and locs, or manipulate their hair to appear kinky—especially those who claim roles as spokespeople or as representatives for these styles, positions from which they profit from Black culture without showing respect for the issues facing Black communities. When I asked Olivia, a 32-year-old Brooklyn resident, who could be natural, she gave a typical response: "White people are definitely not. Some things just aren't for you. Everything else in the world is for you. It doesn't have to be for you. You can enjoy it as well. You are welcome to enjoy it [on Black women]. But do *you* need faux locs?" Here, Olivia decisively argues that naturalness—even artificial naturalness—is for Black women only.

Most white women do not permanently manipulate the texture of their hair, thus adhering to prevailing definitions of "naturalness" as chemical-freeness in the natural hair community. But most of my interviewees decisively positioned white women outside the boundaries of the collective identity around natural hair. Lauren, a 26-year-old woman living in Brooklyn, expressed the broad domain of naturalness while also asserting the political intent of natural hair politics when she told me, "I mean, [white women's] hair is naturally straight. I guess their hair is natural but it's like, less meaningful." While Lauren's statement does not account for the actual diversity in hair texture among white women, it highlights the continuing significance of race in how many Black women understand body politics and the subversive aspect of going natural for Black women. Writer Aph Ko advanced this perspective for the blog *Natural Hair Mag*, writing:

Natural hair was never meant to only focus on texture. It's a political movement that's framed around a particular type of identity resisting white supremacy. To have white women join the movement is counterproductive because they still benefit from white supremacy, regardless of their hair texture.[19]

If natural hair is meant to be a project celebrating Black beauty in a white supremacist society, including white women in the natural hair movement's collective identity, regardless of hair texture, depoliticizes the movement and reinforces the status quo. However, as more Black women embrace their natural hair textures, market imperatives in the fashion industry react by depicting curly and kinky hair as a trend. This is a central feature of capitalism. As mainstream markets attempt to expand, they appropriate countercultural and "revolutionary" styles to sell back to the masses as products of individual self-expression rather than collective critique. Interestingly, despite market conflicts between Koreans and Blacks in the Black beauty industry, as well as a thriving hip-hop culture in Asia, natural hair communities seem most concerned about white women appropriating Black hairstyles.[20] The focus on white appropriation makes sense in societies like the United States and South Africa that are defined by white supremacy, but is also likely because few Asian stars have joined the highest celebrity ranks in the West, and have therefore been less able to materially profit from the appropriation of Black hairstyles.

In the process of converting political symbols into profitable options for self-fashioning, the capitalist marketplace contains rebellious politics. This was the case for the 1970s Afro: recall Corliss, the 62-year-old in Charlotte, and her Afro wig, or activist Angela Davis's lamentation about the "humiliating" reduction of her politics of liberation to a politics of fashion.[21] In the natural hair movement of the 2010s, appropriation and capitalist co-optation continues to be expressed through a push and pull over the racial meanings of curly and coily hairstyles traditionally associated with Black and African peoples, the racial boundaries around natural hair culture, and the limits of fashion. *Allure* magazine's 1970s-inspired tutorial spread "You (Yes, You) Can Have an Afro Even if You Have Straight Hair" (2015) offers an example.[22] The title's additional and emphatic "Yes, You" implies the target audience for the piece: women without the racial, ethnic, or diasporic background referred to by the descriptor "Afro." The article presents the hairstyle as an apolitical trend, featuring a white model, no Black women, and no historical or cultural context explaining the empowering political symbolism Afros had for African Americans during the Black Power and Civil Rights eras. As writer Sherronda Brown explains in an article on why celebrating her Black hair is part of her body positivity practice, "Blackness routinely becomes situated as something which is fashionable when it is taken from us, worn on other bodies. It's a fashion that only Black people are prohibited from wearing."[23] The phenomenon is so widespread that the term "blackfishing" has emerged on social media to describe the trend of white women cosplaying as Black online using image filters, makeup, and hairstyling for Facebook, Instagram, and TikTok likes.[24]

Many have come to view the Kardashian-Jenner family as the epitomic example of "blackfishing," and of the cultural appropriation of Black beauty politics. The celebrity family's position as model appropriators is fueled by their massive influence on the circulation and interpretation of fashion trends, especially in the age of visual social media. Entrepreneur Shantee (42, Chicago) noted, "The standard of beauty today is the Kim Kardashian look. That's what I think our culture is obsessed with." For example, in March 2016, *New York Post* writer Alev Aktar commented on Sasha Obama's cornrows at that year's state dinner:

> The first daughter joins a raft of high-profile beauties sporting a version of the now-ubiquitous boxer braids. Fueled by celebrities and the popularity of UFC fighters, the center-parted reverse French braid style has surged back into fashion. The woven look, dating back to ancient Africa, has been worn by celebs including the Kardashian clan.[25]

Black women, including the young Obamas Sasha and Malia, have been wearing cornrows continuously, long before they were re-popularized by the Kardashians. Shantee observed how pop culture refuses to acknowledge Black beauty unless it is performed on a white body:

> They think behind the scenes that we're beautiful and that's why they steal all of our things, like having a big butt and wearing braids and things that come from our culture. When a Kylie Jenner rocks it oh, it's hot, but when a Black woman rocks it nobody notices. Until Kylie or Kim wears cornrows then everyone wants to rock cornrows but we've been rocking cornrows for how long?

Similarly, after athlete Ronda Rousey wore her hair tied back into two underhanded braids for a fight, fashion magazines began calling them "boxer braids" as if Rousey had invented the style. In reaction to the rebranding of cornrows as boxer braids, Lauren from Brooklyn exclaimed in our interview, "They even changed—it's a new name they are calling cornrows. Like, what is that?" The mainstream media's attribution of cornrows to Rousey is reminiscent of when, in 1980, Bo Derek popularized cornrows for white women as "Bo Braids."[26]

It is undeniable that Black women's bodies are desired by and desirable to whites—the systematic and condoned sexual exploitation of Black women since slavery is evidence of that. But instead of mandating that Black women cover their hair to uphold white beauty standards, as with eighteenth-century Louisiana Tignon Laws, white privilege in the twenty-first century maintains itself through colorblind tactics that adopt and appropriate Black hairstyles without citing their cultural sources. Journalist Kara Brown responded to the boxer braid "trend" on the pop culture website *Jezebel*, writing, "Perhaps Black people would care less about white people taking hairstyles from us, if they weren't also busy taking our lives and basic sense of humanity on a regular basis."[27] These women's reactions frame natural hairstyles, the label attached to them, and the right to wear them as belonging to an in-group of Black women and unavailable to white outsiders. Brown's statement further politicizes the cultural appropriation of Black hairstyles by connecting it to white oppression and the concurrent racial justice conversation around disproportionate police brutality against African Americans. When Solange Knowles released her record *A Seat at The Table* in 2016, it became the unofficial soundtrack of the natural hair movement. The songs "FUBU" ("For Us By Us") and "Don't Touch My Hair" distilled the thoughts and feelings of the natural hair movement into lyrics. The message: Black hair is for Black women—keep your hands off it and off Black women's bodies.

Multiracial African American actress Amandla Stenberg weighed in on the conversation around white celebrity appropriation of Black hairstyles in a video she created as a school project that went viral online. The project, entitled "Don't Cash Crop My Cornrows," (2015) flashes images of entertainers Fergie, Kim and Kylie Kardashian, Christina Aguilera, Katy Perry, and Riff Raff. Stenberg's exclusive use of white celebrities as examples of cultural appropriation frames whites as oppressors and Blacks as the oppressed group, adhering to dominant Black-white racial boundary-making around the natural hair movement's collective identity. She asks the viewer, "What would America be like if we loved Black people as much as we love Black culture?" Her question points to the vast difference between the *performance* of Blackness by celebrities and the *lived experience* of being read as Black in America, a society defined by capitalism, racism, a history of European colonization, and the legacy of slavery. Celebrity appropriation of Black culture is predicated on class power and privilege, as a group of people who not only escape being fired for wearing cornrows or kinky hair, but are rewarded for being creative, edgy, and fashion-forward in doing so—and who return to whiteness when their photoshoots end.

Models, celebrities, marketers, and magazine editors with race and class privilege may understand their appropriation of Black hairstyles as representing a progressive change in racial attitudes and an acceptance or appreciation of Black cultural forms. However, when whites appropriate Black culture without providing a referent or historical context, they "affect a fetishistic 'escape' into the Other to transcend the rigidity of their own whiteness, as well as to feed on the capitalist gains of commodified Blackness."[28] bell hooks further asserts that "when race and ethnicity become commodified as resources for pleasure, the culture of specific groups, as well as the bodies of individuals, can be seen as constituting an alternative playground where members of dominating races, genders, sexual practices affirm their power over in intimate relations with the Other."[29] The revolutionary potential for privileged groups to subvert racist domination by expressing desire for the Other through appropriating the phenotypical signifiers and cultures of marginalized groups is limited, especially in the case of Black hair, since Black women are routinely stigmatized as violent, unprofessional, ghetto, or undesirable for not straightening their hair.[30]

At the same time, a wide range in phenotypes and definitions of Blackness challenge efforts to stabilize a racialized natural hair politics. When *Teen Vogue* prominently featured a model who many readers assumed was white in a feature on Senegalese twists, a style originating in West Africa that is similar to braids, but uses two instead of three sections of hair, the natural hair community on Twitter, Tumblr, and Instagram responded critically. One Twitter user wrote, "@TeenVogue, why's your magazine so anti-Black?????" Then *Teen Vogue* editor Elaine Welteroth defended the article by pointing to the model's Fijian, Tongan, French, English, and American ethnically-mixed roots and connecting them to her own Blackness as a biracial woman. Welteroth's rebuttal to one Instagram user read, "How do you define Black? Just curious. Is it about skin color? Eye color? Hair texture? I ask because this mixed-race model is as Black as I am. Also, how do you define cultural appropriation? I ask only because I want to better understand your point of view."[31] It's unclear from Welteroth's post how she defines Blackness, even as her response reinforced critics' viewpoints that authentic Blackness is a requisite for wearing the hairstyle.

Olivia (32, Brooklyn) expressed this same investment in authenticity while recognizing the difficulty in regulating such a subjective requirement when she told me, "I just think it's like, come from an authentic place. I think you can feel that. I can tell if you're really about that life. It's not really up to me to tell you [that] you can be or you can't be. Just be real. I feel like I don't want to be the natural police because some of the natural police can come at me." As Johnson argues, when something as slippery and dynamic as Blackness is appropriated to the exclusion of others, authenticity can become "yet another trope manipulated for cultural capital."[32] In theory, a focus on authenticity enables marginalized groups to resist oppression and exclusion and police cultural appropriation. In practice, racial authenticity is always at threat of contestation. The difficulty of stabilizing racial boundaries around the natural hair movement demonstrates the limits of collective mobilization when a culturally and phenotypically diverse group bases its racial politics on the body.

Black-led businesses are not necessarily safe from conversations about exploitation and appropriation, as concerns about who owns, who profits, who is represented, and who is encouraged to participate in natural hair spaces can all be at odds with the profit-making pressures of individual naturalpreneurs. Two of the highest profile calls for centering Blackness in the natural hair space responded to companies Carol's Daughter and SheaMoisture's efforts to expand their consumer bases beyond Black patrons. In doing so, both companies were critiqued for capitalizing on the natural hair movement and eroding the Black/white boundaries much of the natural hair movement is keen on upholding. In 2014, African American natural cosmetics pioneer Lisa Price sold her then ten-year-old company, Carol's Daughter, to L'Oréal as profits declined in her New York City brick-and-mortar boutiques. Prior to the sale, Carol's Daughter hired Black celebrities like Jada Pinkett Smith, Solange Knowles, Gabrielle Union, and Mary J. Blige as spokespeople for its promotional materials. After the sale, L'Oréal seemed to abandon the Black-affirming images that had made Carol's Daughter popular. L'Oréal's president Frédéric Rozé explained that the company saw its acquisition of Carol's Daughter as a way to "build a new and dedicated multicultural beauty division."[33] The natural hair blogosphere reeled. From Christina Patrice's point of view in her post for popular natural hair website *Black Girl with Long Hair*, "To allow the brand to fall to the point of being labeled as some bubbling cauldron of ethnically obscure and culturally ambiguous dollar signs and hair milks is an insult to every woman of color who has ever supported Carol's Daughter." Patrice clarifies that, by woman of color, she specifically means "women of the African Diaspora," including those with multiethnic backgrounds. In doing so, she adheres to hegemonic American understandings of Black racial hypodescent and calls for a Black-centered natural hair space.[34]

Likewise, when Bain Capital acquired a minority stake in Sundial Brands, the parent company of the popular natural hair- and skincare line SheaMoisture founded by Liberian-born Black American Richelieu Dennis, it began actively targeting a multicultural audience. A Bain Capital representative told the *Wall Street Journal* that the firm's "investment is aimed at boosting growth by targeting a broader market that isn't defined by ethnicity."[35] SheaMoisture's #BreakTheWalls campaign, produced by marketing agency Droga5, was the first major step to that end. In the minute-long commercial, a group of popular Black and Afro-Latina YouTube influencers with varying hair textures search for products in the ethnic aisle at a grocery store while gazing longingly at the aisle labeled "beauty." There, a blonde, white woman and her daughter, who is only shown from behind but whose blonde coily-textured hair suggests a multiracial background, unsuccessfully search for products. A disembodied voice asks, "Is ethnic not beautiful?" Then, the shelves shake and products fall to the ground, spilling their contents. The commercial ends by announcing that SheaMoisture can now be found in the beauty aisle "where we all belong." In a 2015 Sundial press release explaining the company's partnership with Bain Capital, Dennis said, "I have often said over the last 20 years that the beauty aisle is the last place in America where segregation is still legal and separating 'beauty' from 'ethnic' only served to further perpetuate narrow standards of what is considered beautiful in our industry and society."[36]

Not everyone agreed with Dennis. #BreakTheWalls was met with mixed reviews. Some viewers echoed the sentiment that the ethnic aisle makes them feel spatially marginalized, while others saw the campaign as a naïve move toward colorblindness. Writer Morgan Jerkins penned an article in April 2017 about both SheaMoisture's #BreakTheWalls campaign and the Carol's Daughter sale for the website *Racked* that went viral on social media. In it, she contemplated, "If Black women feel decentered, is the promotion worth it?"[37] SheaMoisture responded to her article on Facebook, pointing out that the company remains primarily Black-owned and emphasizing that they value "listening to underserved consumers (whether the Naturalistas who began with us and empowered women from all backgrounds who now embrace their natural beauty as a result) and delivering on their unmet needs."[38] Nowhere did SheaMoisture racialize who they meant by "Naturalistas." Later that same month, SheaMoisture was shamed again for an ad in their series "A Million Ways to Shea" that featured three white women (two redheads and one blonde) and a light-skinned racially ambiguous woman of color with long spiral curls. Each woman discussed her story of "hair hate" and coming to find "hair love" by embracing her natural hair. Thousands of Black women threatened to boycott the company, accusing SheaMoisture of whitewashing the company's image to expand its consumer base. As Nielsen's 2017 research report on current trends in Black women's consumer behavior explains:

> Black women's values spill over into all the things they watch, buy, and listen to, and while they control the lion's share of the African-American community's $1.2 trillion in spending power, they are doing so with an eye toward the tangible and intangible value of those dollars spent. Black

women not only vote at the ballot box, they vote at the cash register and with their highly influential voices on social media.[39]

Black communities on the social media platform Twitter, collectively referred to as Black Twitter, made "A Million Ways to Shea" a worldwide trending topic that overtook that day's top news stories, including conversations about the looming threat of war with North Korea and Obama's first public event after leaving the White House.[40] Kimberly Foster, the founder of Black feminist website *For Harriet*, denounced the "#AllLivesMatter marketing," tweeting, "Black women built SheaMoisture. And not the 'I was teased for having good hair' Black women. Black women will take it right on down too" (1.5k+ retweets).[41] In an explosion of viral memes, Rachel Dolezal came to symbolize SheaMoisture's use of white women to reconstruct and deracialize Black aesthetic politics. SheaMoisture responded on Facebook and Twitter: "Wow-we really f-ed this one up! Please know that our intent was not, & would never be, to disrespect our community."[42] Notably, SheaMoisture avoided racializing "our community" in their reply to the backlash. Their choice not to acknowledge Black women as their main consumer group highlights deep fault lines between profit imperatives and politics.

The push for Black-centered representation in the natural hair community aligns with the broader political perspectives of the 2010s. Departing from 1990s multicultural appeals for diversity, the natural hair movement often emphasizes the continuing significance of anti-Black racism in determining how bodies are depicted, treated, policed, and disciplined. For example, after George Zimmerman was acquitted for Trayvon Martin's murder in 2012, #BlackLivesMatter formed "in response to the virulent anti-Black racism that permeates our society and to call attention to the ways in which Black people are systematically targeted by state violence."[43] Critics of Black Lives Matter retorted with #AllLivesMatter, and BLM supporters responded by pointing out that Black people are not yet included in the idea of "all lives" having been legally reduced to partial humanity as slaves, presumed violent even when unarmed and laying on the ground, and disproportionately incarcerated.[44] The whitewashing of natural hair discourse is akin to an "All Lives Matter" approach to hair. Just as whiteness shapes ideas about whose lives matter through the repeated exoneration of police officers who murder unarmed and legally-armed Black people, whiteness takes hold of ideas about class and beauty through expectations that Black women minimize and discipline their racialized features to be considered employable, respectable, or desirable.[45] The natural hair movement's investment in defining boundaries around Blackness highlights how post-racial arguments against the continuing significance of race fail to account for the lived and perceived experiences of discrimination women face because of their Blackness, while also striving for representation in the media, for material resources as entrepreneurs and consumers, and for bodily security and respect in everyday life.

The murder of George Floyd by Minneapolis police officer Derek Chauvin in 2020 was an inflection point towards a more mainstream acknowledgement of Black folks' experiences of racism in America both big and small, and the impact of white supremacy on everything from makeup shade ranges at the beauty counter to how history is taught in schools. As protests spread from South Minneapolis across the globe, businesses of all shapes, sizes, and industries finally began to respond to calls for equity in representation, ownership, and opportunity, some with significant resources. Diversity funds were created, donations made, and councils established. As a result, mainstream brands began to include more women of color in advertising, and scores of Black indie beauty brands found homes on big box store shelves like Target and Sephora, allowing more haircare lines that didn't shy away from making products for and marketing directly towards Black consumers to become more easily accessible. In the alternate universe that was life at the height of the COVID-19 pandemic, the capitalist logics that Black-inclusive, Black-centered, and even politicized business won't pay fell apart . . . for a time. Natural hair communities finally got some of what they'd been demanding for years—participation, credit, and acknowledgment.

Interracial Alliances: Colorblind Naturalness

That one of the oldest and most prominent websites for natural hair was founded by two white American women in the late 1990s, years before Facebook existed and blogging became trendy or profitable, complicates attempts to racialize natural hair politics as being for Black women only. I met with Marla, one of the site's founders, to learn how she manages to forge multiracial alliances across the curly hair media and commerce space in the wake of the natural hair movement. By 2017, when the natural hair movement was in full swing, Marla's site reported a global monthly audience of sixteen million readers, ultimately becoming a leading sponsor of natural hair content online. Marla herself has become an influential consultant in the curly haircare market for cosmetics corporations across the globe. Since we spoke, her website has been acquired by a large distributor of beauty products, which uses the site's content to market and measure product uptake in the multicultural beauty space.

Marla's thick, dark chocolate curls rested on her shoulders as she relayed her natural hair journey from childhood to middle age. Her narrative about her natural hair journey helps her justify her right to exist within the natural hair collective space as a non-Black woman. She foregrounds a shared trauma with Black women of not fitting into idealized and restrictive notions of femininity, as well as the struggle to find material and educational resources to care for her hair texture. Her experience aligns with collective identity theory's loophole argument, which explains that "boundaries may be subverted when other axes of differentiation create alternative alliances."[46] "I hated my hair," Marla told me, "and I definitely did not fit into the California look that my peers had." Until she became a teenager, Marla wore a one-inch pixie cut because her mother did not know how to care for her hair texture any other way. "When I finally let my hair grow out, they called me 'Bozo the clown.'" As the years progressed, Marla tried different looks, from ironing her hair into stiff, Farrah Fawcett feathers to applying chemical relaxers that disintegrated chunks of her hair.

In the 1990s, Marla and a friend of hers discussed their mutual struggle to find resources for curly haircare and came up with the idea to start an online message board. With the help of a fourteen-year-old web designer, their site was born. When the natural hair movement gained momentum years after they started the site, Marla and her business partner found themselves in a key position of power and influence. Their site transformed from a simple message board to a company that produces a wide range of online content, retails products, throws festivals, and consults emerging businesses. As the site grew, they struggled to come to grips with a community that was organizing itself around racial politics and Black womanhood. Marla's team responded by featuring more women of African descent, taking classes on white privilege, and providing filters in their online shop to identify both women-owned and Black-owned brands. An article on the site advises white women with curly hair to avoid culturally specific hairstyles, buy products from Black entrepreneurs, acknowledge the specific impact of anti-Black racism, and take initiative to self-educate on racial politics. In doing so, the site's editors recognize the logic and political symbolism of racialized boundaries around natural hair communities while also making space for non-Black women with similar hair textures to participate in conversations about natural hair.

Most often, however, the site's approach to natural haircare evades explicit discussions of race, favoring a texture-first approach. The website helped make popular celebrity hair stylist Andre Walker's Hair Typing System. Walker's original system classified hair texture on a scale from 1 (straight) to 4 (coily). Marla's site added letters (A, B, and C) to further break down the original scale into intermediate categories. A host of bloggers online further extrapolated texture typing to include more than curl pattern: porosity (how well hair retains or releases moisture), density (how close hair strands are to one another), and width (how thick or thin individual strands of hair are). Many people find texture typing useful in customizing their haircare regimens, using the number and letter system to search for bloggers and YouTubers by curl

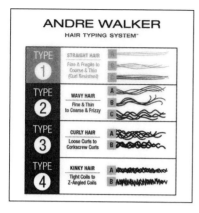

FIGURE 5.1. The Andre Walker Hair Typing System. Courtesy of The Andre Walker Hair Typing System.

pattern and identify techniques, products, and tools to try on their own hair at home.

Hair texture typing discursively makes space for broad, multiple, and multiracial representations of the "natural" body. While most people who participate in natural hair communities identify as Black and have a 3 or 4 hair texture, the acknowledgement of embodied diversity departs from dominant and narrow 1970s views that Black identity or political consciousness is dependent upon one's ability to achieve an Afro.[47] At the same time, hair typing can function as a colorblind system that eclipses the role of race and racism in how hair texture is seen and understood on racialized bodies in social life. Colorblind ideology asserts that racial and ethnic groups are essentially the same despite unequal social locations and distinct histories.[48] In natural hair spaces, colorblind hair typing tends to subtly reproduce a texture hierarchy where looser curls and physical proximity to whiteness are considered more beautiful. The scaled system evokes legacies of good versus bad "grades" of hair. This effect—in a space where many women seek to find resources that re-valuate Blackness—is not lost on Marla's site's readership, and the website's comment sections often become a space for critical exchange. "People write some nasty things in our comment section," Marla told me. She pulled out her iPhone to show me a photo of a very light complexioned woman with

Arab features and waist-length, dark brown, loosely wavy hair that she recently posted on her site's Facebook page. One commenter complained that the subject's hair texture did not represent the natural hair community. Another user retorted that the prior commenter was "just jealous."

This tug of war over inclusion, privilege, and representation personally implicates Marla because she is often called upon to speak on panels at natural hair events and because the site's business model relies on collaborations with Black women entrepreneurs. In our interview and frequently in her public talks at natural hair events, Marla emphasizes that her classmates and sorority sisters were all blonde. By noting hair color alongside hair texture, she acknowledges an Anglocentric beauty ideal without explicitly naming whiteness—astutely positioning herself inside the boundaries of racialized naturalness even though her website frequently features blonde wavy- and curly-haired models. Marla also told me that Black women often enter business interactions with her unsure of her intent and expecting to dislike her on account of her whiteness. "People want to claim things for them, especially when they are not aware of our [website's] history. I didn't come into this to make money. I came into this to provide resources." Here, Marla discursively distances herself from accusations of culturally appropriating Black culture by understating her profit imperative and emphasizing her commitment to natural hair over time. Her statement also recognizes that her right to participate in natural hair movement spaces relies on constructing a multiracial and inclusive collective identity—one that tolerates her whiteness.

Internal Conflicts and Contradictions

Black women do not participate in the natural hair movement with an equal sense of ease, either. This was an issue that I, and many of my interviewees, navigated with varying levels of acquiescence, anxiety, and anger.

Even as authenticity is often put up as a requisite for participating in Black beauty culture and politics, no one can argue that natural hairstyles require naturalness. By that, I mean that much natural hair styling involves using human or synthetic extensions, several layers of styling products, and texture manipulation, like twisting, braiding, or using curlers and perm rods to craft new curl patterns. Many women come to assume that achieving beautiful natural hair requires hard work and consumption, an assumption that is reinforced by an economy of digital tutorials and product review blogs. But the "doing" of natural hair tends to operate in only one direction—toward looser, longer, more defined curls. In contrast to the 1970s, when the natural look meant a round, picked-out Afro, today's natural look favors smooth curls that clump together—a look that some Black women can jump out of the shower with and others cultivate through twisting, braiding, curl-rodding, gelling, and creaming. I fall into the latter category. So, the Thursday before a natural hair event in Brooklyn, New York, I washed and twisted my kinky hair so that it could air dry in time to fall into crisp, frizz-free spirals by the weekend. Sure enough, when I got to the natural hair event, three different natural hair websites and a prestigious national news magazine interviewed me that day—not about my academic research but to feature my "look." The news magazine even invited me to participate in a later photo shoot alongside two Olympic athletes who would compete in the Rio de Janeiro games later that summer. I jumped at the chance, viewing the shoot as an ethnographic opportunity during which I could record field notes in a hard-to-access elite community. I found myself trying to deemphasize my embodied capital by emphasizing my scholarly orientation to the natural hair movement. I eventually ended up discussing my research in an interview with the journalists, but I knew that it was my appearance and not my research expertise that initially afforded me the opportunity to be there. Another time, an entrepreneur I interviewed invited me to participate in a photoshoot after meeting me with my hair twisted. I obliged her, rationalizing my acquiescence as an effort to reciprocate the time and trust she dedicated to my work by sharing her story with me. I mention this experience to prove an uncomfortable point: the natural hair movement is most welcoming to people who look like me—women who can accomplish long, loose, curly styles and still be seen as decidedly Black.

As a researcher, I found that whether I could achieve my goals during fieldwork depended on how I looked that day and how "polished" my hair was.[49] As I reached the saturation point in my research process I discovered that my hairstyle and attire tended to facilitate or shut down my conversations with other attendees in the field, so I made a habit of writing preliminary field notes on my appearance. If I wore my hair in braids, a head wrap, or in a "wash and go" with my unaltered and tightly coiled hair texture, I faded into the background and was ignored for hours at a time. However, when I manipulated my hair to mimic a looser curl pattern, I had much more fruitful interactions with research participants, and most people assumed my twisted hair grew with that curl pattern because my hazel eyes and medium-light brown skin tone suggested some sort of mixed ancestry somewhere in my family history. But I'm also easily read as Black, and like other women with similar phenotypical characteristics, my right to participate in natural hair spaces and the categorization of any manipulated hair style I wore as "natural" were never questioned.

Curls Are the New Kinks

Two decades prior, I likely would have gotten very different reactions to my appearance as an ethnographer studying this topic. In the 1990s, sociologist Shirley Anne Tate found that the light-skinned and multiracial women she interviewed in her study on Black beauty politics dis-identified with their embodied privilege as they critiqued other Black women for straightening their hair, wearing weaves, or otherwise taking "unnatural" steps to appeal to a white aesthetic. She argues that multiracial women's dis-identification from their privileged positionality is triggered by shame and melancholy about their distance from the politicized Black beauty ideal of dark skin and tightly-coiled hair. However, this ideal has shifted since the moment in which Tate collected her data. The women in Tate's study were reacting to the political legacy of the 1970s "Black Is Beautiful" era, when the ability to achieve an Afro was viewed as the benchmark of ethnic legitimacy and "the Blacker the berry, the sweeter the juice" was a common refrain among Black folks. In contrast, the natural hair movement of the 2010s prizes curls rather than kinks. Corliss gestured to my twist out in our interview to explain the difference between the Black beauty ideal of the present moment and the Black beauty aesthetic of the 1970s: "People are not just wearing Afros. They wear it like you and curly. People would wear puffballs then, but they weren't like you. They weren't curly."

This new ideal may be influenced by the fact that two of the earliest brands catering toward naturally curly hair textures to find mainstream success were developed by multiracial Black women who created products based on what worked for their hair textures. Mixed Chicks and Miss Jessie's images of silky, cascading curls formed the bulk of natural hair representation in the 2000s and early 2010s. In the years that followed, most natural hair products similarly aimed to reduce frizz, combat shrinkage, define curls, and perfect twist-outs. Now, mixed-race Black beauty is no longer outside the bounds of politicized Black beauty, and instead, it has become the ideal form of racialized natural beauty. Fannie, a natural hair expert in Los Angeles who travels internationally to present at natural hair conferences, observed of the natural hair movement: "They like the light-skinned curly mixed look. It's exotic to them. They really do like light-skinned, curly-hair girls. That was just because we were trained not to like our Blackness."

Media studies scholar Meeta Jha notes a resurgence of colorism in her analysis of the shift and commodification of anti-racist Black beauty aesthetics since the 1990s.[50] She argues that the current idealized image of political Black beauty is contradictory and best symbolized by performer-entrepreneur Beyoncé, who approximates many aspects of white feminine beauty ideals—long, blonde, usually straight or wavy hair—while taking advantage of being racially perceived as Black to sell herself, Black culture, and feminist empowerment at the same time. For example, in the music video for "Formation," (2016) the Black girl power call for solidarity, Beyoncé sings, "I like my baby heir with baby hair and Afros" while she alternates between a curly, blonde lace-front weave that drapes to her mid-back and blonde braided extensions. Kristin Rowe notes how Beyoncé destabilizes the cultural reverence of white women's bodies in *Lemonade*'s "Sorry" with the line "You better call Becky with the good hair," publicly articulating a shared sense of embodied intimacy among Black women who have been othered for not measuring up to Eurocentric standards of beauty and heterosexual desirability.[51] Yet, Beyoncé maintains her signature long blonde look three years later in "Brown Skin Girl" (2019), a song celebrating the beauty in the diversity of Black and Brown women's skin tones. While women in the video don a wide variety of hairstyles from closely cropped "teeny weeny Afros" (TWAs) to meticulously-crafted braids, all of Beyoncé's own looks feature either long or loosely textured styles. In her debut advertising for her and her mother Tina Knowles' haircare line Cécred in Essence, Beyoncé dons both long, blonde, loosely braided spiral tendril curls and bone-straight looks. When asked who Cécred is meant to serve, Beyoncé responds that the product collection intends to show that "any textured hair could be healthy"—a lesson she learned at her mother's salon.[52] In doing so, she celebrates the creative possibilities of hair play, emphasizes her personal history as the daughter of a Black hairdresser, and avoids alienating anyone. Just as Beyoncé simultaneously embodies resistance and conformity to racialized beauty standards to be marketable, so does the natural hair movement. Both are invested in Blackness but struggle to keep those most marginalized at their center.

Trading in on Texturism

As I did the research for this book, I observed as many natural hair influencers followed Beyoncé's path, elevating to positions of power in natural hair spaces precisely because they fit into the ideal of light-to-medium complexioned skin and long, loose, "natural" curls. For example, a popular mixed-race woman in her late twenties who I'll call Monet catapulted to natural hair influencer status based on her appearance. I had seen Monet's famous blonde curly halo and heard about her in interviews years before I met her. Fannie, the hairstylist I introduced above, explicitly used Monet as the example of the prized "exotic" look and a public figure many women "freak out" over. Monet's influence reached so far and wide that Marlene, a 45-year-old teacher living thousands of miles away in Cape Town, confessed to me in a whisper that she follows Monet on social media, but that Monet's apparent happiness, beautiful hair, and toned bikini photos make Marlene feel ashamed, inadequate, and irrelevant as a middle-aged woman. Three months later, I met Monet at a technology and music conference that hosted a natural hair meetup that reported over 4,000 attendees. Monet was a featured panelist who discussed her natural hair journey alongside five other natural hair influencers. The event coordinator moderated while Monet's friend videotaped her responses on Snapchat and Instagram live from the first row. Monet sat cross-legged on a director's chair dressed in a black lace mini-dress and thigh-high suede boots, sandwiched between a natural haircare product entrepreneur and a popular natural hair website owner. By coincidence but not unnoticeably, the panelists were arranged by skin tone from darkest to lightest. Monet explained that around three years earlier she casually took some photographs with a friend. When Monet posted them on her personal Instagram page, natural hair websites and their associated social media accounts copied and saved her pictures, which they likely identified through the natural hair hashtags she used in her captions. By reposting them on their own Instagram, Twitter, and Pinterest pages, these natural hair accounts disseminated Monet's image to their thousands of followers without her explicit consent. Many of these accounts tagged her personal page, leading Monet to amass over 330,000 Instagram followers by 2021. She eventually became a highly sought-after speaker at natural hair conferences around the world. Monet has since capitalized on her appeal by becoming a full-time brand ambassador for many high-profile fashion, hair, and travel companies and blogs. All of this ensued without any initial intent of becoming a natural hair blogger and without any specialized knowledge about haircare. During her talk at the tech conference, Monet stressed the importance of having a likeable personality in her advice to prospective bloggers in the audience, emphasizing that looks are not enough to maintain an engaged following. Indeed, natural hairstylist Fannie said of Monet, "She's just a pretty girl anyway so people love her and she's sweet." Accentuating likability, especially to an audience diverse in phenotypes and age, acts to restore a sense that a career as a natural hair influencer requires merit and that texturism does not discount the effort that conventionally beautiful women expend to maintain their status and celebrity.

Many women I spoke with pursued and banked on the privileges of looser curls, albeit uneasily. Through trial and error with her look over ten years of auditioning, 30-year-old Hollywood actor Aaliyah was acutely aware of the social and material privileges loosely curly natural hair affords Black women, especially as mainstream media embraced the natural hair trend in the mid-2010s. Aaliyah has a deep brown complexion and describes her hair as a tightly coiled "4C,"[53] but she successfully booked three national commercials with a curly weave that was less coarse than her natural hair texture. Her weave shifted how people interpreted her deep brown complexion, almond-shaped eyes, and overall racial-ethnic background. She noted, "everybody likes to throw out the exotic word . . . people would ask me, 'oh your hair, your eyes, what are you mixed with?'" She scoffed, rolled her eyes and replied to me in proxy, "I'm just mixed with Northern Black and Southern Black." Over time, Aaliyah became disillusioned with the entertainment industry's partial acceptance of Black beauty and her acquiescence to a mixed-race Black beauty ideal. Speaking about her weave, she explained, "I just want to be me, and I'm just at a place where I'm just done faking it you know?" She continued:

I don't think some people would dispute the fact that we live in a country that has conditioned us to hate the part of us that's African ever since we got here and you know there have been points in history where I think like Black beauty has been like celebrated but it's a certain type of Black beauty. It's certain, like, body features so I just don't want the uphill battle I have to fight with raising a child that is half Black and half something else and then me having to teach them that this something else doesn't make you more beautiful because the person who is 100% Black is beautiful, whatever 100% Black means. You get what I'm saying, the person who's 100% white is beautiful. Our differences make us beautiful, but you're not more beautiful because your hair has a looser curl or because your skin is light or your eyes are lighter or that doesn't make you more beautiful. But I feel like, I don't know man, we live, we live in a world where it's like you go to a school and there's a whole bunch of different kids in a classroom, you know. Nobody's walking up to the Black girl with like short braids or pigtails telling her how beautiful her hair is, but people are going to do it to the kid that's mixed. And I think, I just, I've always wanted to raise Black children to be proud of who they are no matter how they look. And you know, if it happens for me and I end up, you know, having mixed kids so be it. But I just feel like I have to fight a little bit of an uphill battle in terms of, you know, making them really be proud of being Black because they're going to be taught it's the other part of them that makes them more beautiful.

Aaliyah includes mixed-race women within the bounds of Black identity and Black beauty, recognizing that "100% Black" is neither a stable nor useful requisite for a racialized beauty politics. At the same time, Aaliyah notes how texturism and colorism continue to marginalize darker-skinned women and girls, including her own natural beauty. A few months after I interviewed Aaliyah, she shaved her head, ended her career as an actress, and left Hollywood for seminary. Her decision reflected her inability to reconcile her pursuit of unconditional Christian self-love with demands from her agents that she de-emphasize her racialized features to become more commercially marketable in the entertainment industry.

Ambivalence, Anxiety, and Anger: Finding Where You Fit

Sociologist Maxine Craig notes that overt colorism and straight texture privilege have always been a source of debate within Black communities.[54] During the Black Power Movement, artists and activists widely and publicly challenged these pressures in iconic pieces like Toni Morrison's novel *The Bluest Eye* (1970) and Spike Lee's film *School Daze* (1988), which portray the emotional and social destruction color and texture competition produces among Black women. Recent documentaries *Dark Girls* (2011), *Light Girls* (2015), and *Hair Tales* (2022) have revived conversations about beauty politics and colorism in Black America, portraying how color-based stereotypes hurt all Black women, albeit in different ways, and also what individual hair stories reveal about Black innovation, resilience, and creativity. Women in the natural hair movement have heard—and felt—these critiques and contradictions. Almost every person I interviewed expressed an acute sensitivity for colorism and texturism in the natural hair movement community and in Black culture more broadly, even if they stood to profit from these hierarchies.

Shantee, a natural haircare business owner with light brown skin and waist-length spiral curls, wrestled with her own aesthetic privilege in representing her company. Since she was a child, Shantee dreamed of being a hair model like the little girls on the *Just for Me* relaxer box. But paradoxically, Shantee hated being heralded as the "pretty girl" with light skin and long hair among her peers in middle and high school because she felt that such comments undermined and dismissed her experience with racism as a Black girl. As an adult, Shantee made her childhood modeling ambitions come true by serving as the spokesperson for her own natural haircare company. During our conversation, she expressed her continued ambivalence to the exclusionary light-skinned beauty ideal by instructing her social media staff to "post all different hair textures and hair types and skin colors because we feel that's a better representation of us." Shantee's business exclusively posts women and girls of African descent on its Instagram account. However, her followers are quick to push her to center not only Blackness, but dark-skinned beauty. Shantee's voice quivered when she told me:

> I've noticed that when we post someone that is light-skinned and a looser curl pattern we'll get comments that say, 'well you guys never post anyone with 4C hair or a tighter curl pattern' and we could just have posted someone with a tighter curl pattern five minutes ago . . . we constantly want to tear someone else down. I get it, too. People want to argue me up and down and say that you're not Black. You're not fully Black because you're light-skinned and your hair is long. How come I can't be fully Black? Because I'm light-skinned with long hair? It is hatred in our own race.

Her response highlights that the division and hurt texturism and colorism cause operates in multiple directions. While few question Shantee's right to participate in natural hair politics, her elevated position within natural hair spaces and her right to represent her own business are constantly up for debate. But, Shantee's testimony shows that women privileged by hair type can and do strive to use their influence to actively prioritize diverse representations of Black women.

Olivia, a 32-year-old, mixed-race light-skinned woman I interviewed Brooklyn also feared capitalizing on colorism to sell a magazine she founded to cover Black beauty and the natural hair movement. She attempted to remove her body from view entirely—not just on the pages of the magazine but also behind the scenes, and initially searched for a dark-skinned business partner who could serve as her company's public spokesperson. She explained her rationale during our conversation:

> I know that my experience is very different than other experiences and I don't think it's the most important . . . It's still like being light-skinned with

curly hair is more acceptable. Putting a darker brown skinned woman on the cover with [an] Afro is more of a statement. It means something, and not only that but it speaks to women who are so often ignored and it's just like, I don't want to talk about myself too much. I want to do something bigger and greater for people who are way too often written out of the conversation.

Olivia eventually decided that she had the right to speak in natural hair spaces upon considering how slavery, Jim Crow, and anti-Black discrimination have affected her and her family's history, as well. She pulled up screenshots of old sepia-toned photographs of her mother as a child riding a horse in their poor and working-class Midwestern neighborhood: "They grew up with nothing really, in the country too . . . That's the stock I'm coming from on my Black side. I think we all have a strong sense of being Black American and that if you are here today you have survived some craziness and you are strong." She justifies her right to participate in Black politics in general, and natural hair politics in particular, by pointing toward the lived effects of race and anti-Black racism on her family. Reflecting on her initial ambivalence in starting an endeavor in the natural hair space, she told me, "There's a definite difference [in how my hair is perceived] but that doesn't mean we shouldn't have a dialogue and we can still find beauty in each other. Me feeling like I couldn't voice that you are beautiful with your natural hair—I'm entitled to that too." In her view, her personal, familial, and historical experiences of racial marginalization authenticate her right to express a Black-affirming beauty politics as a light-skinned and mixed-race woman. Zaire (23, Los Angeles) similarly pointed to a lived experience of Blackness when she told me:

Some people who are a few shades darker than me feel like they've earned their Blackness. I don't think the tone of my skin determines whether I'm Black or not, like my features, my family, the texture of my hair, everything that I've known is living the life of a Black person. I wouldn't be able to attain the privilege that white people have so no matter how much people jokingly or being mean try to tell me that I'm not Black, there's nothing else that I can be.

Since women are often blind to each other's personal histories, and since hair textures are so relative, diverse, and malleable, hair is a medium through which women in the natural hair movement continuously construct and deconstruct extremely complex identity politics over and against one another. As image activist and former fashion editor at *Essence* magazine Michaela Angela Davis summarized in *Light Girls*, "Black women have been cultured to compare, not connect."[55] Constant assessment of skin color, hair texture, and phenotype creates situations where emotions run high, and boundaries around who can and should represent naturalness feel fraught. For example, once, at an event on natural hair held at a Black history museum in Los Angeles, a group of elderly African American ladies dismissed me from their conversation about the significance of the natural hair movement, asserting that I had no understanding of the pain of Black hair. "Look at you," they simply said, and swiftly ended our conversation. I turned away without comment, because I understood their desire to privilege their own experiences as senior women who navigated decades of intensely hurtful colorism, and I knew from experience that my voice in natural hair spaces was granted more attention and power when I looked the way I did that day—young, able-bodied, lighter-skinned, and with my hair styled in a twist-out. I also could sense that we were all feeling too sensitive for our discussion to have a chance at making it past skin deep.

Worries about where one fits within the natural hair movement often precede transitions to natural hair, especially since many new naturalistas have never seen their hair texture as adults. Some women evaluate the possibilities and outcomes of their and other women's decisions to transition to natural hair based on the "goodness" of that person's hair texture. For example, Corliss told me about a conversation she had a week before our interview, where a friend told her she "had a nice grade of hair, so when it grows out naturally it is going to be beautiful." The remark gave her confidence to continue her transition, but it's easy to imagine the damage a different assessment could have done.

Since many of the most famous natural hair influencers have silky, curly hair, lots of women feel anxious about discovering a hair texture that looks like the bloggers that they follow for inspiration and encouragement, and are disappointed if they discover themselves outside of idealized "natural" beauty. In an article for the natural hair publication *CRWN* magazine, writer Candace Howze describes a similar experience, writing:

> As I excitedly watched my own curls emerged, I decided they were a tight 3C. I couldn't wait to have bouncy S-curls popping loosely from my head. However, when I big chopped in February 2015, something wasn't quite right. My hair was not 3 anything, except for the soft patch near the nape of my neck. It was all over 100% Type 4 and I was shocked. Terrified. Shamefully disappointed . . . The main reason I went natural was because I wanted to know what my real texture was, what the real me looked like. But now, I just felt disappointed by the truth.[56]

Howze's discovery that her natural hair texture is more tightly coiled than those she follows on social media had a politicizing effect: "This sobering revelation opened my eyes to an issue we must overcome: texture discrimination and representation."[57] Michelle (49, Los Angeles) describes her own hair texture as a tightly coiled 4C or 4B; she explained her reluctance to compare her own hair texture with influencers in the natural hair blogosphere when she told me:

> There's a girl Naputral85 and another girl MahoganyCurls. You can just tell they have a different texture of hair. They're mixed with something and no matter what they do with their hair it's going to curl up and give them the best twist-out and the best whatever . . . I don't want

to be in a conversation where everyone's just like, "Oh, you've got good hair." It shouldn't be that conversation.

Several women with tighter textures or no curl pattern have been vocal about the impact of texturism on their experiences of having natural hair and of the natural hair movement itself. In an article for the *Huffington Post*, Zeba Blay describes her personal struggle to love her kinky hair texture despite her political commitment to its anti-racist symbolism, blaming colorism in the natural hair community. She appropriately observes, "the politics of [natural] hair don't necessarily escape the influence of white beauty standards."[58] For example, mega-popular beauty blogger and influencer Taren Guy publicly critiqued a natural hair expo on social media for canceling her as a speaker after she abandoned her long, bouncy curls and started the process of transitioning to freeform locs. She discussed her experience in a caption on an Instagram post:

DEAR NATURAL HAIR COMMUNITY: Transitioning into locs has really shown me the tremendous love and vulnerability that women of color posses [sic] with words of support, wisdom, relatable testimonies and hopefulness of one day letting go of those things that keep them from moving forward in their truth. I've also experienced the B side of the online natural hair community that I was aware of but still sort of blind to. A side that has truly turned this beautiful space into a commercialized industry. My locs haven't even been a week old and I've already been canceled for a NATURAL HAIR event due to my hair change as it "doesn't fit the demo and audience of the attendees" nor does it sit well with sponsors. I'm a bit disappointed, not because I won't be attending, but because a space that was created to empower women of color with ALL types of natural hair has turned into a show that only support one type of natural. This post is not meant to be negative . . . It's just real. And it's a problem. Shout out to all of the beautiful women out there who celebrate their uniqueness while empowering and supporting women trying to do the same . . . Women who are keeping this beautiful space alive with the intention to educate, inspire and express themselves freely![59]

The cancellation of Guy's speaking engagement demonstrates one way that texturism and capitalism mutually reinforce one another—by excluding certain bodies from representation and economic opportunity.

Some Instagram and Tumblr accounts dedicated exclusively to celebrating women with kinkier textures and increasing their representation in the media and beauty industries have become grassroots subcommunities within natural hair spaces. These groups create new collective identities framed both by race and texture, and they may have real impact on how some women see themselves. Tina, a 25-year-old high school teacher, told me she follows dozens of dark-skinned women she's never met on social media to boost her own self-esteem as a deep-complexioned Black woman with tightly kinky hair. She credits these accounts for inspiring her choice to abandon synthetic twists and to loc her own hair. Sherronda Brown penned a separatist 4C movement manifesto in response to SheaMoisture's "A Million Ways to Shea" commercial. In it, she declared: "This movement is for and about the people with the type of hair that shrinks all the way up to our ears, like the way this society demands we shrink our Blackness for the comfort of others."[60] Preferring the term "negro hair" to "natural hair," Brown discursively emphasizes Blackness in rewriting desirability politics, and calls attention to body size and facial features as additional axes of exclusion within natural hair representation. Even still, Brown acknowledges that she is often asked what she's mixed with and told she has good hair, despite that she identifies as a "type 4" natural.

"It Would Have Been Okay to Create an Exclusive Space": Fragile Boundaries in South Africa

Color and texture conflicts were particularly salient among women I interviewed in South Africa, as hierarchies within the natural hair movement uncomfortably mirrored hierarchical racial boundaries between women of African descent. In South Africa, there are four main racial categories: Black, Coloured, Indian, and white. Black is used to refer to the country's population of indigenous Sub-Saharan Bantu-speaking tribes, while Coloured is used to refer to the population of multiethnic descendants of European colonizers, sub-Saharan African tribes, indigenous Khoikhoi and San tribes, and formerly enslaved people from Southeast Asia. The apartheid government constructed Blackness and Colouredness as mutually exclusive, and Coloured South Africans received preferential treatment in jobs, prisons, hospitals, and schools. Coloured people's hair textures range from *gladdes* (straight/sleek) and *krulle* (curls) to *kroes* (kinks)—often with wide variance among families—while most Black South Africans have very kinky hair. Wearing one's natural hair texture undermines the blurry boundary between Black and Coloured because the groups' hair textures overlap. 26-year-old Raven from Cape Town explained, "When it comes to hair, having your hair in this [natural] state is degrading, basically, because it looks more like the next Black person's hair. It doesn't look like the next Coloured person's hair or the next white person's hair. For Coloured people, being whiter is better but being Black is a downgrade." Brie, also from Cape Town, concurred, "I find that the majority of Coloured people I know highlight their European ancestry rather than the Khoi San or the Indigenous side of us." No person was ever legally reclassified from Black to white during apartheid, but some Coloured people successfully legislated their way to whiteness through the "pencil test" that rewarded *gladdes* hair.[61] The cultural significance of hair texture in the Coloured community is evident through insults like *bossiekop*, an Afrikaans term that translates to "bushy head" in English, used to tease and bully Coloured women with kinky or tightly coiled hair.

As an intermediate group in an apartheid racial hierarchy that privileged whiteness and denigrated Blackness, Coloured people have stood to gain more socially, politically, and materially by appealing to white aesthetic ideals and distancing themselves from Blackness. But, for several Coloured South African women I spoke with, transitioning to natural hair was a pathway to embracing a Black identity and possible African ancestry for the first time. For example, Raven grew up in an exclusively Coloured community and never met or communicated with any Black South African people until she went to college in her late teens. Upon being misread as Black by others with her newly natural hair, Raven began to identify as Black in addition to Coloured. She told me:

> I consider myself Black actually. Because I have such a distorted background of my family tree, I'm not quite sure if I might have some Black genes in me. As far as I know, both of my parents are Coloured, but I have features that look Black so I have started becoming more conscious . . . I just feel like I can relate. I have started reading the likes of Oliver Tambo and Steve Biko. I'm reading them now for the third time because every time I read it, it speaks to something different in my life.

Coloured and Black women participate in the same natural hair movement online and in event spaces, which tend to de-emphasize or ignore racial differences to create cohesive communities that focus on self-esteem, styling, transitioning, and coping with kinky-curly hair stigma. Many Coloured and some Black South Africans understand crafting a multiracial natural hair collective as a strategy for deconstructing Black-Coloured distinctions rooted in South Africa's white supremacist European colonial history. However, enduring texture hierarchies subtly reinforce the apartheid racial order and complicate alliances between Black and Coloured women, who are more likely to have looser curls. Sheila, a Black South African woman living in Johannesburg, explained how texturism exacerbates preexisting racial divides when she told me:

> There's that debate about the goodness of your hair. Your hair is good because you're mixed. Its less coily if you're mixed so there's that thing that oh, well, you're mixed so it's not that natural. It is natural *but*. It's

a natural *but* if you didn't have white blood in you it wouldn't look like that. So, there is that debate. It goes deep. There's always that what do you call it? A clash between the races about what is natural and what should it look like and that's where the Coloured and the Black will then come in.

Most influential bloggers in Cape Town's natural hair scene are Coloured women with long, silky, defined curls. Several Black South African interviewees expressed disappointment that a Coloured student of Black and Indian descent became the symbolic figure of the protest at Pretoria Girls High School against white-centered school grooming policies, despite the fact that the protest was organized by a mostly Black collective of students. Sheila observed:

> You see the Pretoria Girls issue if you see who is in the forefront . . . It's the *girls* that are experiencing the struggle not a *single* girl but now they've changed it to be about this girl. That's the type of girl they would go for because the other girl is not good enough. Her hair is not good enough. You don't have the good hair therefore you don't fit the mold.

Texturism in South Africa's natural hair movement can often feel like the reification of apartheid racial hierarchies that privilege Coloured women over Black South African women.

Some Black women I spoke with felt that Coloured women appropriate Black African hairstyles, like Bantu knots, and should form separate natural hair spaces to mitigate hurtful distinctions between "good" mixed hair and "bad" Black African hair. Stacey (29, Cape Town), a Black South African woman of Kenyan descent, rationalized:

> For Coloured women especially, the battle around hair is big for them too. I feel that it is good that they are doing this but I kind of feel like they should acknowledge the people that started it and it would have been okay to create an exclusive space. I think we struggle to acknowledge

these differences and dark-skinned women bear the brunt of it ... It's one thing for a whole group of women to be erased because we just don't have any of these appearing white, closer to white features, and to know that and then to have someone who is, whose hair is less kinky. Whose hair makes a prettier Afro because let's face it, all the Afros we say we like are these loose bouncing Afros."

Stacey's statement highlights the broad appeal of natural hair politics for women of African descent living in former European colonies. Her position also aptly emphasizes how local and relative racial understandings, hierarchies, and histories shape whether the natural hair movement's aesthetic is experienced as reproductive or resistant. For example, a suggestion that multiracial women take initiative to form a separate natural hair community in the United States would be taboo against the backdrop of brown paper bag tests that barred darker-skinned Blacks from elite social organizations in the Jim Crow era.

Lindi, another Coloured woman from Cape Town, resented the idea of separate Coloured and Black natural hair spaces, arguing that her curly hair texture and multiethnic background should not exclude her from a Black identity and do not produce a less meaningful experience of transitioning to natural hair:

[Coloured people] always sitting in the middle of it. We sat in the middle with apartheid and we are sitting in the middle now. With apartheid job preference went to us first and we got looked down at from our Black brothers and sisters. I want to break divides. I want to break down that wall and break down that barrier because I look at myself as Black. Don't get me wrong in saying that I am proud to be who I am. I am proud of who I am. Our history is big, its massive, but it includes Black people and it includes white people as well so why isn't that okay? Who says that it wasn't as hard for you to actually make the move to return to natural? I had this conversation with someone I call a friend and she said it's really great that you have decided to do this but we need to get our kinkier curlier girls to do this as well. What about my story? Yeah, but you weren't really pointed at school. Bull! Yes I was. Absolutely! I was. I was called a *bossiekop*. I was told please do something about your hair because you're natural. I went through hell. Don't make it as if what I went through is less than what you've went through because you've got a thicker texture. Embrace yourself. That's all.

Lindi's statement acknowledges the Coloured community's privileges over Black South Africans during and after apartheid, while challenging the notion that Blackness and Colouredness are mutually exclusive identities. Lindi notes her white ancestry, but she does not claim whiteness. Instead, she emphasizes Black and Coloured women's similarly painful experiences of not matching up to white-centered beauty ideals in a society slow to dismantle its recent history as a white racial dictatorship. Perhaps Lindi's suggestion to work toward self-love is the best chance for overcoming the divides created by texturism and colorism within natural hair spaces across the globe, since each person's subjective experience of "hair hate" and "hair love" is never fully knowable to others.

Conclusion

So, who can be natural? This question preoccupies natural hair spaces, and yet the boundaries around natural hair politics continue to be messy and unstable. The constant negotiation of who can wear natural hairstyles like braids, weaves, twist-outs, and Afros and the political meanings associated with them, documented here, illuminates the character of twenty-first-century social justice agendas, wherein anti-racist social movement communities of the 2010s favor Black-centered and race-conscious strategies to combat anti-Black racism. Returning to the opening example of this chapter, writer Ijeoma Oluo's analysis of her interview with Dolezal for the *Stranger* succinctly summarizes many Black women's view on the political nature of Black feminine embodiment:

> Even if there were thousands of Rachel Dolezals in the country, would their claims of Blackness do anything to open up the definition of whiteness to those with darker skin, courser hair, or racialized features? The degree to which you are excluded from white privilege is largely dependent on the degree to which your appearance deviates from whiteness. You can be extremely light-skinned and still be Black, but you cannot be extremely or even moderately dark-skinned and be treated as white—ever.[62]

Oluo argues that the wholesale exclusion of Black women, both light-skinned and dark-skinned, from whiteness and white privilege requires a necessarily exclusionary Black feminist collective identity if Black feminism is to subvert white supremacy. Similarly, natural hair communities are largely protective of natural hair as a project specifically of and for women of African descent, a project that makes claims for social recognition, and for expanded concepts of attractiveness and professionalism, which have historically privileged white middle-class femininity. Wearing kinky and curly textured hair has become a symbolic celebration of Black beauty and a form of activism that aims to *reorganize* and *redistribute* resources—representation in the media, market share, employment opportunity, access to healthy haircare, aesthetic and cultural value—along intersecting race and gender lines. In doing so, women of African descent have produced new knowledge and ways of caring for their bodies, and have given new, politicized meanings to the kinky textured, braided, and twisted hairstyles that they've claimed as their own. Including non-Black women in natural hair representation is often likened to reducing the anti-police brutality campaign Black Lives Matter into a colorblind "all lives matter" image. Given the long history of racial conflict over Black hair's political symbolism and market share within the "ethnic" haircare industry, centering women of African descent in natural hair politics has become a political and moral priority for many.

Fannie, a hairstylist from Los Angeles, summarized dominant sentiments when she reflected, "The only way that Black lives will matter is if we stop spending money in communities that aren't ours." The racialization of natural hair's collective identity, while fragile and challenging, remains an important mobilization strategy for combatting anti-Black gendered racism in the United States and beyond.

Yet, the descriptor "natural hair" does not overtly connote the racialized image that many naturalistas intend. Black women's efforts to create representational and affirming spaces for themselves require that they construct a boundary around the natural hair movement's collective identity that frames them as an oppressed group fighting for representation and cultural credit. This boundary requires constant maintenance, especially as market interests routinely threaten to depoliticize natural hair's anti-racist symbolism and market it as simply one of many trends to try. Many beauty and haircare companies project a colorblind, multiracial vision of natural hair that downplays different racial histories and the privileges of proximity to whiteness to appeal to the broadest possible consumer base and to sell as many units of product as possible. Likewise, as the fashion and entertainment industries take notice of more Black women embracing their natural hair textures, journalists, stylists, and editors interpret kinky hair and braids as edgy trends open to anyone for the taking. In doing so, these industries neglect the cultural and historical significance of hair and hair texture for women of African descent. As with many other consumer-based political projects, global capitalism does its best to absorb and profit from the natural hair movement's grassroots community.

Many women of color understandably experience advertisers, celebrities, and mainstream corporations' colorblind representations of natural hair culture as co-optations of a movement they feel is political. To reassert the political intent of the natural hair movement in a neoliberal capitalist moment that celebrates self-fashioning and choice, some Black consumers actively reassert boundaries around a collective identity they claim as their own. As I've documented here, communities of Black women use the language of cultural appropriation to call out fetishistic and exploitative adoptions of Black hairstyles and movement discourse, deeming white women as inauthentic outsiders and Black businesses attempting to racially diversify their consumer base as shameful sell-outs.

To complicate things, Black identity itself is diverse, shifting, and variable from place to place. This diversity challenges the radical intent of an embodied Black feminist identity politics. Texturism and colorism continue to hierarchize Black women's "natural" beauty in societies founded on white supremacist ideals. This issue is clearly observable in advertisements and in the upper echelons of the beauty influencer community, where women with lighter skin and looser hair textures receive the most attention and opportunity. It has become a source of deep hurt and anger that darker-skinned women and women with tighter coils remain underrepresented and stigmatized within natural hair communities. Black women with highly textured hair, especially those with darker complexions, are unequivocally justified in their critiques of the natural hair movement's exclusionary ideal that subtly privileges proximity to whiteness. How can those who are invested in centering Blackness practically and responsibly deal with difference? I believe that natural hair politics can avoid essentializing Blackness or reviving regressive blood quantum debates among Black women by foregrounding the *experience* of racial marginalization through hair texture. Sociologists and race scholars Omi and Winant warn us that racial projects become racist when they rely on essentialist logics, or the idea that cultural groups are naturally and intrinsically different from one another.[63] The idea that race is biological and unchanging unproductively asserts that those with relative power and privilege are unable to understand or empathize across race and color lines. After all, some white women, like Marla, can and do endeavor to work alongside Black women without culturally appropriating Black hair and its political symbolism. Moreover, most light-skinned women I interviewed, like Olivia and Shantee, are sensitive to their color and hair texture privilege and actively prioritize inclusivity. Yet for the natural hair movement to really help liberate Black women in a capitalist, patriarchal, and white supremacist society, community members must always be mindful that they act within the social relations and from the subject positions we wish to change. Even the most well-meaning advocates can't separate themselves from the cultures in which they live.

What's a more effective way of thinking about who can be natural? Crafting a beauty politics that's more than skin deep. A collective identity that emphasizes a shared subjectivity and advocates for non-comparative self-love while recognizing and actively counteracting social hierarchies and their impact on representation offers the best chance for overcoming the divides created by texturism and colorism within natural hair spaces. A greater acknowledgement of the emotional, cultural, and structural influences on embodiment can push us past the dichotomous and oppositional mind-body divides inherent in Western thought, while also encouraging respectful empathy and compassion for oneself and for others. Sociologist and Black feminist Patricia Hill Collins's conceptualization of the Afrocentric notion of beauty, which includes mind, spirit, and body as simultaneous factors in theorizing aesthetics, is a helpful starting place.[64] What did hairstyling mean for your ancestors, and how has that impacted you? What did the spectrum of representation in children's books, magazines, and on TV teach you about the worthiness of your own body? What thoughts, emotions, and dilemmas arose when deciding how to wear your hair for school pictures, weddings, and job interviews? Have you ever had to rediscover your hair? Was it by choice, what did that feel like, and what did you learn? Imagine the opportunities for sisterhood, understanding, and solidarity that might arise by tackling these questions together and taking seriously what we hear.

Conclusion

Detangling Texture

Over the course of the 2010s and into the '20s, the natural hair movement has traveled through Facebook groups, expo halls, city parks, college chat threads, YouTube channels, salon suites, and living rooms across the African diaspora. Many of you might have been part of this wave yourselves, grappling with what your transition to natural hair meant in an intimate sense: to your bodies and its wellbeing, or to your self-image and self-esteem. This book aimed to show that the personal is also very political by addressing four questions: Why are Black women around the world organizing around the idea of naturalness, and what does naturalness mean to them? What makes natural hair a movement, and how does it fit into Black women's calls for social change? What do natural hair politics reveal about today's gendered racial boundaries, hierarchies, and conflicts? How is the natural hair movement reorganizing Black women's relationships to the Black beauty industry, the global market, and each other?

The natural hair movement has brought attention to texturism as a social issue within and beyond Black communities, one that underwrites how Black women experience embodiment at their intersections of race and gender. In this book, I have described how the natural hair movement has enabled some women of African descent to reimagine their beauty, over and against controlling images of Black bodies in general, and Black hair in particular, as wild, unprofessional, ugly, or unfeminine. Naturalness, as a descriptor of unstraightened curly, kinky, and coily hair textures, leans on the idea of authenticity to re-valuate Black women's physical qualities and traits. As the women of the natural hair movement embarked on their personal journeys of transition and texture rediscovery, they created alternative images, practices, and products that celebrate curly, coily and kinky hair. Their representations, advice, and reflections circulated in digital spaces and inspired a worldwide shift in beauty culture. In turn, women of the natural hair movement expanded their possibilities for consumption and entrepreneurship and challenged the racial order of the beauty industry, which had not well-recognized natural Black beauty or served Black women's unique needs and experiences. The movement's emphasis on body autonomy and the right to take up space found its way into broader environmental and anti-racist social movements in ways that assert intersectionality, making Black women's experiences of racism legible to those in power and to others in their communities.

Black women have done all this social and political work against the odds. Disparaging comments by television pundits, family members, and coworkers—in addition to racist, sexist, and texturist institutional grooming policies—continue to pressure women of African descent to change their appearance in favor of a white, middle-class beauty ideal for long, straight hair. And while hair straightening can be a mindful and strategic practice to ensure upward mobility through employment or the dating markets, many women I met expressed having internalized the patriarchal and white supremacist messages from the media, their families, and coworkers that lighter skin and long, straight hair are more beautiful, more professional, and more feminine. Most women of the natural hair movement chose natural hairstyles despite holding such beliefs, and they continue to encounter the effects white supremacy within natural hair spaces, where colorism and texturism cause hurt, hierarchy, and division.

The stories of the women in this book reveal new insights about how race works, and how the body is a medium between and productive of racial consciousness and social racial identity. While the sociology of race tends to focus on bodies simply as racial signifiers, by focusing on texture, I have tried to show that bodies have a much greater role in racialization and racial politics. Race, I argue, is also created, invoked, obscured, and reimagined through the self-representative choices people make. People can and do express, emphasize, or minimize their identities through choices like hairstyle, fashion, makeup, plastic surgery, and the way they carry themselves—often in politicized ways. For example, I introduced multiracial interviewees in South Africa and Brazil who embraced a Black identity for the first time due to their transition to wearing their natural hair texture—a theoretically significant pattern that highlights how embodiment can be a third strand in the interplay between identity and social norms that seek to impose the value of racial categories from the top down. As women of African descent style their hair with attention toward respectability, resistance, or authenticity, they show how individuals have agency in how they navigate social structures. Black women's bodies—before and after their transitions to natural hair—are both the product of capitalist, white supremacist, and sexist systems *and* people's responses to and experiences of those systems. In other words, bodies are simultaneously objects of and agents for racial formation. If we only consider how macro forces represent and categorize race, and fail to recognize how individual people shift their self-representation and self-identify at the micro-level, we miss out on an entire dimension of how race can be, and is being, critiqued, reworked, and reimagined.

This book also challenges common feminist assumptions in beauty studies about the (lack of) potential for consumer-based politics to contribute to meaningful social change.[1] Most of that research describes women who feel pressured to purchase goods and services like plastic surgery, skin-lightening creams, diet regimens, and fitness programs to adhere to a sexist and narrow beauty norm while feeding the capitalist machine. Women's experiences of and agency within beauty cultures are often omitted from these critiques of neoliberal beauty. By highlighting the subjective experience of Black women's beauty work, I have showed that natural hair can be both political and transformative, in spite of and *because of* its consumer capitalist orientation. The rise of web 2.0

technologies alongside natural hair politics has enabled some women of African descent to circumvent retail and distribution systems that have historically excluded Black folks through emergent online retail storefronts, natural hair meetups, and influencer blogging and vlogging communities. The natural hair movement of this century, like Madame C.J. Walker's fleet of pressing comb saleswomen of the last century, has produced *more* possibilities for a Black middle-class through additional modes of entrepreneurship. Naturalpreneurs, with their intimate knowledge of caring for textured hair, are reclaiming expertise, re-entering the Black beauty industry, and recirculating profit within their communities. Many of those I interviewed exemplified possibilities for pushing against the unfair economic, political, and industry structures they work within, challenging the ways most scholars have understood the characteristics, scope, and outcomes of capitalist politics, beauty politics, and identity politics. Moreover, organizing around a new definition of naturalness—one that foregrounds integrity and authenticity in addition to texture—shows how neoliberal, biomedicalized frameworks can create productive opportunities for care and critique. Today's naturalness borrows frameworks from the green movement to politicize wellness, self-care, and self-love as ways of "doing" Black feminism. Their experiences and outcomes suggest that neoliberal capitalism is not monolithically negative for Black people, but diverse and potentially unexpected. And so, researchers should not take for granted how race, gender, culture, and social location shape experiences of and responses to neoliberalism, or what communities stand to gain through engagement with its pressures.

Though biomedical discourses of self-scrutiny often serve the interests of global capitalism, and though class continues to stratify who has access to natural hair discourses and healthy products, it is also important to note that many naturalpreneurs actively engage Black working-class communities in ways and to depths that environmental feminists, regulatory bodies, and large retailers have not. For example, upon struggling to find affordable natural hair products in her area, Paula (27, Los Angeles) created her own low-cost natural product line. She describes her business as "a means to an end . . . an end to being anything but completely and wholly without boundaries—boundaries put on us by society, by time, and by money." Naturalpreneurs like Paula have made careers brewing organic and ethically-sourced hair potions to sell to health-conscious women in their communities, while influencers like Whitney White, who shares do-it-yourself alternatives to packaged products, market a "green" hair politics. In the process, they advance precautionary care and consumption as a Black feminist wellness project. I also attended natural hair meetups where organizers pushed to secure greater access to healthy foods in low-income areas, advanced literacy in evaluating the toxicity of chemicals in cosmetic and food products, and connected natural hair politics to other causes like mental health and breastfeeding. Nonprofits like Black Women for Wellness educate at natural hair events. To summarize, though natural hair culture operates within the flows of neoliberalism, it does so in ways that promote not just individual body projects, but also collective efforts of health promotion in response to decades of unhealthy personal care practices grounded in gendered racism. More wellness activists should consider using salons, cosmetology schools, natural hair events, and online natural hair forums as sites for public health advocacy. This could do crucial work, since much recent medical research links chemical relaxers to various reproductive health illnesses that Black women disproportionately experience.[2] We need more interdisciplinary and intersectional research on the relationship between beauty ideals, beauty practices, and health disparities.

While much research has focused on Black women's exclusion from representations of beauty in western mainstream media in a general sense, less work has discussed how Black women in unevenly-developing countries like South Africa and Brazil are further marginalized within diasporic Black spaces that are, in theory, globally accessible in the digital era. This book has tried to emphasize the importance of social and historical context for what beauty, politics, and beauty politics mean. When broadening from a focus on the United States, it becomes apparent that global political and economic arrangements stratify women's access to power within the natural hair movement. While Black American women live at the bottom of race, gender, and often class hierarchies in the United States, they are privileged by their status as *Americans* living in the developed Global North. Black American natural hair influencers and entrepreneurs dominate the global Black haircare market and the production of natural hair culture, spreading many American-centered frameworks, as evidenced by analogies between #AllLivesMatter and #AllCurlsMatter.

American hegemony, global capitalism, and white supremacy intersect to constrain the possibilities for cultural production and consumption in much of the Black Atlantic. In Canada, South Africa, Brazil, the Netherlands, France, and Spain, almost all products for Black consumers available in beauty supply and convenience stores are not only made for straight hairstyling but are manufactured by American companies. Even though African American naturalpreneurs struggle to compete in a hostile and exclusionary beauty market at home, they benefit from American cultural and economic privileges abroad. Women living in the United States are overrepresented in the natural hair blogosphere, and the content they produce casts American products as must-have "holy grails" while ignoring the fact that most American-made products are inaccessible to or prohibitively expensive for the rest of the African diaspora. This affects market demand abroad. On several occasions, potential interviewees for this project in South Africa negotiated for samples of American natural hair products as compensation despite affordable, effective, and accessible alternatives manufactured by local businesses. This sort of African American cultural imperialism also shapes women's natural hair organizing efforts outside of the United States. The first natural hair organizer in the Netherlands told me that she started a company importing hard-to-get American natural hair products. She then began hosting natural hair events to teach her customers how to use them.

Not all of the naturalistas I met outside of the United States welcome or idealize American influences. Some women explicitly acknowledge and work hard to counteract unequal global relations within this diasporic cultural movement. In Cape Town, I sat in on a meeting of a collective of natural hair bloggers and business owners as they strategized against rumors that companies SheaMoisture and Cantu had contracts with major South African convenience stores in the works. These entrepreneurs were highly aware that a sole emphasis on Black representation in the natural hair movement ignores intersecting social positions like class and global location that privilege some Black women over others in an unevenly globalizing world. South African naturalpreneurs worried about their livelihoods, and they pointed out that their needs would continue to be unmet by the American market due to differences in climate, hair texture, and cultural tastes. I had much to learn from these women's perspectives, and I strived to remain wary of imposing my own Black American perspectives in conversations like this. I was again reminded of the importance of reflexivity and positionality when an American entrepreneur I interviewed, whose products focus on "mixed" naturally curly hair, explicitly described South Africa as a new frontier for her business to conquer. It was clear to me that she did not realize that Coloured people do not think of themselves as "mixed-race" in the same way some multiracial Americans do, nor was she considering Coloured people's experiences of forced removal and segregation from both Black and white South Africans. It worried me that she spoke of her business's mission that way because it resembled a sort of economic imperialism that further disrespected local histories, challenges, and racial relations. Future researchers might further probe how global inequality stratifies other efforts at diasporic and pan-African politics, collaborations, and cultural exchange.

Future Directions in Black Beauty Studies

There's so much more to learn about beauty within the African diaspora, and so much to further understand about the ways in which Black women's positions within and experiences of beauty culture differ across the Black Atlantic and vis-à-vis one another. Since I was interested in theorizing natural hair politics as a gendered racial project and a potential form of Black feminist resistance, I chose field sites with similar histories of European settler colonialism and slavery. Though women in this study share a political reality and embodied experience under white supremacy, I hoped to also show how local contexts and global power hierarchies shape what naturalness means in different parts of the Black Atlantic. But this research cannot predict or generalize about what natural hair means to all women of African descent, because our histories are much too varied. Future research might further investigate what contemporary natural hair cultures on the African continent might reveal about globalization, cosmopolitanism, ethnicity, and identity in the digital era, especially as new natural hair salons, online forums, and meetups are proliferating all the time in places less defined by racial difference, including in Kenya, Nigeria, and Ethiopia.

In addition to exploring the expanding dynamics of diaspora and transnationality, future research should also take gender identity as another lens through which to analyze Black beauty politics. This research cannot begin to make claims about hair for all Black women, as the natural hair movement spaces I encountered during my fieldwork rarely foregrounded queer experiences. And yet, Black queer communities have always been innovators in Black beauty culture as they shape, reimagine, and reconstitute beauty norms. Styles of wigs and weaves, as well as the language of "beat" faces or "slayed" looks all originated in Black queer and trans spaces, and now they're all part of the mainstream aesthetic cultural and lexicon. Black queer femmes are often the makers of taste, techniques, and terminology that push global culture forward, and all the while, queerness compels us to reconsider what femininity is, means, and looks like. How are dilemmas around commodification, individual empowerment, collective racial uplift, appropriation, authenticity, and respectability further complicated when Black queer and trans women's experiences with hair are foregrounded? I look forward to much more research and writing in this area to come.

And, while beauty studies primarily centers femmes as subjects, Black masculinity has its own storied hair history. Past research has examined barbering as a trade that allowed many Black men to circumvent the pitfalls of a racist job market,[3] but intersectional scholars have less-widely applied a lens of embodiment to men and their relationship with hair. Such research is incredibly timely, sociologist Kristen Barber points out, because neoliberal pressures are compelling men to participate more deeply in beauty culture.[4] How is this reconstituting, reinforcing, and expanding Black masculine norms? Understanding these tensions and possibilities is central to theorizing beauty politics for all Black people.

Finally, it is important to note that this book reflects the unique moment in time during which I was in the field—the mid-to-late 2010s—ending just before the onset of the COVID-19 pandemic. The pandemic profoundly transformed society in numerous ways, including its impact on beauty practices among Black women. As lockdowns and social distancing measures were implemented globally, many individuals adapted their beauty routines to accommodate remote work, virtual interactions, and reduced opportunities for in-person socializing. With salon closures and limited access to professional services, some Black women embraced DIY approaches to haircare and skincare, experimenting with new styles and products at home. Others likely reevaluated the emphasis on external appearance in light of the pandemic's toll on mental health and well-being, prioritizing self-care practices that nourished the mind, body, and spirit. Additionally, the heightened awareness of systemic inequalities and racial injustices brought about by the pandemic and the murder of George Floyd took conversations about redefining beauty standards and embracing authenticity and self-love beyond niche communities. This complex interplay of factors underscores the need for future research to explore emerging beauty practices among Black women in the post-pandemic era, shedding light on the intersections of race, gender, culture, and resilience in navigating societal challenges with ever evolving resources and worldviews.

Lessons and Legacies

> who's gonna make all
> that beautiful blk / rhetoric
> mean something.
>   like
> i mean
>   who's gonna take
> the words
>   blk / is / beautiful
> and make more of it
> than blk / capitalism.
>   u dig?
> —Sonia Sanchez, 1970, "blk / rhetoric"

What legacy will the natural hair movement leave? Perhaps we can look to the past and its impact on our present for some insight. In 1970, after a decade of organizing around Black Power, poet and activist Sonia Sanchez wrote the poem "blk / rhetoric." In it, she commands and demands meaning from Black rhetoric—the symbols and cultural artifacts of Black folks. Sanchez recognized that the "blk / rhetoric" of natural hair and the message of "Black Is Beautiful" could just as easily fall to the whims of trends, commodities, or catchphrases as they could rise to become heroic calls for change. In response, Sanchez encouraged the Black community to make full use of Black culture to subvert white supremacist capitalism. Reading her work fifty years after its publication, I can't help but wonder if Sanchez is either prophetic or simply an observant student of the waxing and waning of sociocultural movements: The Afro of the 1960s and 1970s was depoliticized, Black-owned businesses were bought out, and mainstream media co-opted Black Power's resistant symbolism. As a child of the 1990s, I encountered more Afros in costume sections of Halloween stores than I did in my community. But despite the historical lesson of the Afro, I am optimistic about the potential for this natural hair movement to create lasting changes in society and on Black women's lives.

Since many women I met align their transitions to natural hair with other transitions to exercise, holistic wellness, green personal care, and healthy eating, I expect natural haircare practices to be just one aspect of Black women's enduring lifestyle changes. As I discussed in Chapter 3, naturalness has assumed new definitions in the twenty-first century alongside a burgeoning green movement. "Natural" has become descriptive of both hair texture *and* the integrity of ingredients in haircare products. This multifaceted definition of naturalness is the distinguishing feature of twenty-first-century Black beauty activism. And, unlike the mainstream environmental justice movement, natural hair spaces are centrally concerned with the particular and intersectional environmental risks Black women face. Thus, the implications of the natural hair movement are more than ideological; the natural hair movement has become an intersectional public health project that fills gaps left by governments, mainstream corporations, and activist groups, which have long neglected Black women's needs by focusing on more privileged groups and more publicly-visible environmental issues.

Structural changes are also arriving in the form of new protections for Black women at work. In June 2019, California made headlines for passing the Creating a Respectful and Open World for Natural Hair (CROWN) Act, which prohibits the denial of employment and educational opportunities because of hair texture or styles like braids, locs, twists, or Bantu knots. The passage of the CROWN Act is incredibly crucial for the protection of working-class women, who have less agency and power to advocate for their freedoms at work. The Act is the result of the energy and momentum built when the CROWN Coalition, a partnership between the National Urban League, Color of Change, Dove, and the Western Center on Law and Poverty, helped amplify grassroots calls for change that had been percolating for almost a decade in natural hair forums, meetups, beauty shops, and family rooms from Los Angeles all the way to Johannesburg. By the time the federal bill was introduced to the US House of Representatives in March 2021, Colorado, Maryland, New York, New Jersey, Virginia, Washington, Delaware, Nevada, Nebraska, Oregon, Illinois, and Connecticut had passed similar laws in their states. With over 500,000 signatures on the official petition to make the CROWN Act federal law, pressure for this kind of legal protection for Black women seems like it could bear fruit soon.

But alas, our Black feminist godmother Audre Lorde reminds us that we can't depend on the masters' tools to dismantle the masters' own house.[5] Since much stigma against locs and Afros still persist around the world, and as texture hierarchies continue to loom large, I expect that many Black parents will continue to worry that their children's hair styling choices will undermine their chances at school, on the job, and in relationships. Already in Texas, a judge has ruled that a school district's dismissal of a Black male student for long locs did not violate the CROWN Act, illustrating how narrow, white-centered constructions of masculinity have begun to erode the spirit of the law and demonstrating how men are facing increasing pressure to adhere to aesthetic norms.[6] And, as naturalistas and naturalpreneurs strategically downplay color and texture differences within the natural hair community to optimize their marketability, color- and texture-blind racism will continue to threaten to depoliticize and individualize the natural hair movement.

I hope that inner healing and this new natural hair movement's politics of authenticity will endure what Sanchez calls the "quick fucks" with white power—in this case, shifting style trends, institutional policies, and market changes. After all, the women I interviewed describe finding a greater sense of self-acceptance and self-confidence through the experience of transition, such that they feel they have more agency and confidence to explore natural hair, straightened hair, weaves, braids, and coils alike and as they desire. As I write this final chapter in 2024, I am observing more open, curious, and vibrant online conversations among Black women about tradeoffs between time, affordability, convenience, pride, and health in choosing hairstyles—conversations not framed in dichotomous terms of "good" vs. "bad," or "conscious" vs "self-hating."

I, for one, find that to be an expansive form of progress, and moreover, I've become one of those women. I don't feel any less authentic, feminist, or anti-racist when I press my hair; rather, I feel as if I'm enjoying the rewards of a decades-long movement that allowed me to see, feel, and act upon a sense of bodily autonomy. I find myself enjoying a less heavy, more playful, and more thoughtful relationship with the way I treat my body, in general. An ongoing commitment to wellness, empowerment, and freedom has shaped not only my choices in hair and beauty work, but other areas of my life as well, including nutrition and childbirth.

It is inevitable that the new natural hair movement, like all moments in Black beauty history and all racial projects, will be but a moment in time. But if, as a result of the new natural hair movement, we can get to a point where "all that is important is [ourselves]," we get closer to *the* point of it all: that Black bodies matter—kinky, curly, straight, weaved, shaved, braided, loc'ed, light, dark, and all. Women who participate in the natural hair movement broadly describe and experience natural hair as an intimate project of self-love, self-care, and self-confidence—a politics of authenticity despite pressures that they change their bodies to appeal to externally-defined Eurocentric and patriarchal norms. Going natural produces new knowledge—new ways of thinking about self and society—that foreground Black women's subjectivity. Though misogynoir remains alive and well and attempts to govern all our choices, I hope and expect that the natural hair movement generation will teach their loved ones to say "I'm beautiful" to their reflections in the mirror, "don't touch me" when touch is unwanted, and "I belong here" anywhere they go.[7] That, I hope, will make all this beautiful "blk" rhetoric mean something.

ACKNOWLEDGMENTS

No research is an independent venture. A great deal of thanks is due to the many people and communities without whom this research would not have been possible. There would be no book without the generosity of my interviewees and research participants. To all those who trusted me with discussing the most intimate of subjects—their bodies—I owe you an immense amount of gratitude. I hope these pages fairly honor the playfulness, pain, passion, adventure, and beauty of your experiences.

All the research and most of the writing that went into this book took place while I was a student at the University of Southern California, where the Department of Sociology and the Program for Women's and Gender Studies supported my work. I could not have completed this book without the mentorship of Michael Messner, Elaine Bell Kaplan, and Lanita Jacobs. Mike's thoughtful feedback greatly broadened how I think about bodies and social movements, and I'm a much more thoughtful sociologist for it. Likewise, Elaine's commitment to the grounded theory approach was central in moving me beyond the insights of existing literature, and closer to the meanings women create in everyday life. Her encouragement to take a stand in my writing gave me the moxie to go against what the canon assumes, and to stand firm that Black women's standpoints matter. Finally, I am so appreciative of Lanita's mentorship as a pillar in the scholarly literature on Black women and beauty. It means so much to have someone who understands and appreciates the value of research on Black communities, especially in a discipline where such work requires constant defense. Lanita's detailed and generous notes and her presence as a role model are central to this work. I am also grateful to Pierrette Hondagneu-Sotelo, Sarah Gualiteri and Leland Saito, who nurtured me as a theorist, and supported my early work.

Many other scholars have read and helped improve my writing, among them Kit Myers, Michela Musto, Jeff Sacha, Jennifer Candipan, April Hovav, Robert Chlala, and Nathaniel Burke. My friends and sister scholars Carolyn Choi and LaToya Council deserve a special thank you for being my sounding board and academic confidants. Carolyn has seen this project develop from the very beginning and fed me—literally and figuratively—with home cooked Korean food, sisterhood, and creativity. From Hollywood School to the CLC Collective, Carolyn constantly reminds me that our work as women of color studying our own communities has real-life implications and that we should never undervalue or ignore our aspirations to become scholar-activists and public intellectuals. Thank you for being a colleague and a friend. LaToya Council, thank you for generously reading my working papers and being my partner in sociology for the fifteen years.

While at USC, I was also lucky to be supported by the loving staff in the Sociology Department, who became like mothers to me. Amber Thomas-Handford allowed me to sit at her feet in her office, sometimes for hours at a time, to talk out my ideas about life and work. Stachelle Overland fought for me and my research countless times, reminding me of my strength and purpose as a Black woman in academia. Melissa Hernandez and Lisa Losorelli also made the research possible. These four women have been such blessings in my life.

I have also been amazed by how many institutions believed in this project. The United Negro College Fund/Mellon Mays Undergraduate Fellowship provided me early mentorship and research training. Spelman College professors Cynthia Spence, Zandra Jordan, and the late Bruce Wade helped me see a path for myself as a scholar. The Social Science Research Council and the Del Amo Foundation supported travel for my fieldwork in Spain and France, as well as my participation in the Black European Summer School in the Netherlands. The USC Center for Feminist Research provided grant assistance for my participation in the

De-Colonial Black Feminism Summer School in Bahia, Brazil, where I collaborated with researchers and activists across the Black Atlantic who contributed to my theorizing.

Many thanks are owed to Ilene Kalish, my editor at NYU Press, who was supportive and enthusiastic about this project from the very beginning. I am also grateful to her assistant editors, Yasemin Torfilli, Priyanka Ray, and Sonia Tsuruoka, and the entire editorial board who helped make this project possible. I also thank the several anonymous peer reviewers for NYU Press who gave me valuable feedback on earlier drafts of this book. Also, Shelby Brewster helped me navigate the many technical aspects of publication with grace and patience, and Dolma Ombadykow's meticulous notes were invaluable in the home stretch. Finally, it was such an honor and a full circle opportunity to have had Paula Champagne, my dear childhood friend, illustrate the cover of this book. Her creative brilliance makes holding this book feel so much more special for me, and I'm especially grateful that this project reunited us.

I am further indebted to my village for holding me up and holding me down as I completed this work. My friends Savanna Ramsey, Raven Evans, Kimberly Mayo, Rebecca Rougeau, Aisha Benton, Kovie Biakalo, Ziyanda Kenya, and Su Jan Chase deserve all the love for sticking with me, checking in on me, and celebrating every milestone along the way. An extra special thank you to "The Clover," my Spelman sisters Nia Newton, Melina Zúniga, Blaire Spaulding, and Ashley Martinez. These women are daily reminders of the power of sisterhood. I love you each, and I love us.

Finally, my family has been unconditionally supportive of me and my scholarship. My mother's decades of activism and advocacy made room for my personal and professional journey to Black feminism, and as a result, this book. I am also thankful for the men in my family—Paparuu, Alan, and Brian—who were quick to forward me any natural hair article, social media fiasco, or magazine spread they came across. To my husband, Jonathan Rabb, I do not take it for granted that I live life alongside a person who supports my scholarship regardless of whether my research makes life inconvenient or uncomfortable. Jonathan was present for two full years of my fieldwork, traveling across the country and internationally as I raced to events and to meet interviewees. He spent many hundreds of hours next to me in coffee shops, motivating me to just write one hour longer, and talked out my findings with me most evenings. Thanks for believing in me enough to join this ride.

APPENDIX A

Researching Bodies in My Own Body

Feminist research does not purport to be neutral. It has become standard practice in feminist ethnography for the author to provide a biographical account of the experiences that drive their interest in the research, and how their positionality vis-à-vis research participants and sites affect data collection and theorizing. Importantly, I share many experiences with my interviewees, including transitioning out of chemical relaxers, resistance toward natural hairstyles by family and romantic partners, and dealing with comments about my hair in my professional environment. I have been a consumer of imported human hair, worked to revalue the physical traits that signify my Blackness, and resisted the ways I have been presumed incompetent in my predominantly white professional environment because of my hairstyling choices. I have had my hair searched by officials at the airport for contraband, by strangers to satisfy curiosity, and by both bullies and intimate partners for proof that it is "real." I have also sat at the feet of other Black women in college dorm rooms, swap meets, expos, salons, and kitchens, bonding with these sisters over beauty work. Thus, I began this project with an intimate awareness of common Black American haircare practices and a familiarity with colloquial terminology used to refer to common African American hair textures, technologies, and techniques.

Because I relate personally to this topic, I employed the reflexive dyadic interviewing method,[1] which encourages interviewers to share their personal experiences, reflections, and feelings with interviewees to open conversation and minimize power imbalances between researcher and participant. As with much feminist ethnography, my participants and

I often discussed the ways in which our life experiences aligned or diverged. We played with those ideas, theories, and hypotheses together. Interviewees were curious about the themes that were emerging during my research process, and I often spoke with them about my findings and whether they held true to their own observations. The public excitement around natural hair was so great that I was asked to write several articles for publication in popular media outlets while I was in the field.[2] Natural hair culture is lively on the internet and propelled through content creation, so these articles were disseminated widely across social media networks. Because of the nature of social media, interviewees and online commenters became active participants in my theorizing process. This meant that I was always accountable to my collaborators, as interviewees and as audiences spoke back to me about what I was finding, seeing, and saying. I constantly felt the pressure that anthropologist Lanita Jacobs describes to "get it right."[3]

Even though I shared axes of identity and experiences with some interviewees, my status as a researcher always separated me from them. My main motivations for entering conversations and attending events were unusual, and sometimes people noticed that I moved around spaces differently. My graduate student status seemed to help my ability to recruit and sustain relationships because many people I met expressed pride in my academic pursuits as a young Black student and considered speaking with me as a contribution to my education and to racial uplift more broadly. But, I always needed to establish trust with interviewees, since it is often difficult to reflect on something so personal as the body and beauty work. There were interviews where I could not establish the rapport necessary to overcome the awkwardness of a tape recorder sitting visibly between my interviewee and me. For some interviewees, I sensed that speaking to me felt especially risky if they had read my public sociology about hair online, in a context where everyday women become mini-celebrities as online influencers. I intentionally negotiated power relations in these situations—and I often failed. I reiterated to participants that I would not disclose any of their identifying information and that I was held to strict ethical policies and procedures as a university researcher, but this simply emphasized my disproportionate power as the person holding the pen. In these instances, we unfortunately remained trapped in an unfair and unproductive power dynamic.

At first, I sought to fade into the background during fieldwork; however, I was repeatedly compelled into more interactive participation through questions about my own appearance and presentations-of-self both in-person and online. This is a common experience among beauty researchers. For example, Mears, Kang, Jacobs, Banks, and Weitz each describe how they and their research assistants were explicitly and implicitly "read" by other women in the field.[4] I moved through events and spaces with a distinct feminine gender identification, age, racial and ethnic identity, class background, and nationality that at times hindered and at times facilitated fieldwork. Realizing that I cannot step out of my own body, I actively embraced the ways in which engaged participation enhanced my data collection. I got into the habit of recording descriptions of my appearance and attire each time I entered the field and before interviews to help contextualize my conversations with participants. I became more of an "observing participant"[5] who was actively engaged in my surroundings, rather than a participant-observer who distanced herself from action in the field.

Depending on my styling choices, I often ended up on the interviewee side of conversations by being mistaken for a natural hair influencer—an elite social actor in the natural hair scene whose career involves providing beauty advice and product reviews. The more work I put into my appearance by washing my hair ahead of time (a two-day task), putting on makeup, and dressing fashionably, the more eagerly fellow attendees interacted with me. In other words, my styling choices affected my positionality. My hair texture, hairstyle, skin tone, eye color, makeup, and outfits were often called into dialogues, usually to acknowledge my mixed-race background. This pattern inspired Chapter 5, which discusses intra-racial color and texture hierarchies within the natural hair movement. For example, at one natural hair expo, I got into a conversation with Debra, a brown-skinned fitness blogger who looked to be in her mid-forties, as we waited for a hair fashion show to begin. In complimenting me on my hair texture, Debra asked, "Are you mixed?" I told her no, and that although there are multiple ethnicities on both my mother and father's side of the family, we all consider ourselves Black. I showed her pictures of my mom and dad on my iPhone. Debra said I look just like my dad except for my eyes. I decided to push the envelope a little bit and told her that my mixed-looking features were the result of rape by slave masters and not of love, because this is true. Debra replied, "Well at least you got something out of slavery!" While Debra said this jokingly, our interaction still highlights the continuing significance of colorism and texturism, or proximity to phenotypical whiteness, even within a movement to re-valuate Black beauty. In Chapter 5, I include more of these auto-ethnographic anecdotes to describe how color and texture hierarchies and boundaries operate within natural hair culture and complicate notions of solidarity. While these interactions were often uncomfortable for me, they were also analytically helpful by illuminating how women interpret beauty ideals and police racial authenticity among and in relation to one another.

My positionality during fieldwork and interviews outside of the United States was complex, but facilitated my research in some interesting ways. For example, in the South African context, I was most often read as Coloured as opposed to Black South African because my hazel eyes and medium complexion suggested a multiracial background. Being read as Coloured by Coloured South Africans often created a sense of openness to critique the Black-led political process in post-apartheid South Africa and the resulting policies and cultural commentary that saturate mainstream media outlets. At the same time, Black South Africans expressed a level of cultural and experiential solidarity with me as a Black American with a lived understanding of anti-Black oppression in the United States context. Phenotypically and culturally straddling the Coloured and Black racial categories in South Africa seemed to facilitate meaningful conversations with people who identified with either group.

Conversely, my American privilege challenged some interactions and data collection outside of the United States. One situation is worth highlighting here for its theoretical and methodological significance to this study. Several South African participants asked me for American product samples as compensation for interviews, probably because there happened to be a Black American filmmaker in Cape Town at the same time I was, who was interviewing women for a documentary about Pan-Africanism and hair, and who recruited interview participants with product samples from a leading American beauty company. This created a moral dilemma for me, because my conversations with South African business owners made me hyperaware of how uneven power relations in the global beauty market privilege American corporations and Black American culture. I feared participating in and perpetuating this situation to the detriment of local business owners. I decided that the best thing to do was talk about it. I met with the American filmmaker, and we had a tense but fruitful conversation about the global, economic, and cultural implications of our recruitment tactics. We mutually decided it felt unethical to disseminate American products to benefit our own work, and discussed the situation together with a South African natural hair blogger on a radio show, and separately, with several Cape Town natural hair entrepreneurs who generously allowed us to sit in on their group meetings while they strategized the creation of an online hub to connect local bloggers with local businesses.

In sum, the results of academic research go beyond the final product of a publication. Theory-making always has an impact, and that impact is more than theoretical. Our activities, our bodies, our decisions, and our indulgences and divulgences are active variables in the field, and they have real and material consequences for the communities we study. As a Black feminist researcher, I aimed for my impact through this project to be as intentional, responsible, accessible, and equitable as possible.

APPENDIX B

Information on Interviews

TABLE A.1. Descriptive table of participants

Sample characteristics		Naturalista (consumer)	Naturalpreneur (Influencer, business owner)	TOTAL
		(n = 62)	(n = 17)	(n = 79)
Location				
United States		44	10	54
	California	23	3	26
	Florida	2		2
	Illinois	1		1
	Indiana		1	1
	Louisiana	1		1
	Minnesota	1		1
	New York	10	3	13
	North Carolina	4		4
	Pennsylvania	1		1
	Texas	1	1	2
	Washington, DC		2	2
South Africa		11	4	15
	Western Cape	7	3	10
	Gauteng	4	1	5
Europe		6	2	8
	Spain	2	1	3
	France	3		3
	Netherlands	1	1	2
Brazil		2		2
	Bahia	2		2
Age				
	18–29	25	6	31
	30–39	20	5	25
	40–49	13	3	16
	50–59	1	2	3
	60+	3	1	4

(*continued*)

TABLE A.1. Descriptive table of participants *(continued)*

Sample characteristics	Naturalista (consumer)	Naturalpreneur (Influencer, business owner)	TOTAL
	(n = 62)	*(n = 17)*	*(n = 79)*
Gender			
Men		9	9
Women	62	8	70

BLACK HAIR GLOSSARY

AFRO *n.* A hairstyle in which kinky or tightly curled hair is combed out to form an evenly rounded, cloud-like shape. The hairstyle became popular among African Americans in the late 1960s and early 1970s, when Black Movement communities presented the style as signifiers of Black pride and appreciation for Black beauty.

BAD HAIR *adj.* A term in Black culture used to describe very tightly coiled hair. Synonyms include *nappy* or *nigger hair.*

BIG CHOP *v.* A form of transitioning where a person cuts or shaves the entire head to immediately remove hair. Most often used to remove permanently straightened due to chemical relaxers, heat styling, or another damaging process. In some rare but highly publicized cases, natural hair influencers have filmed second big chops of their natural hair to resist perceived over-attachment and an excessive identification with their long hair.

BRAIDS *n.* Hair that is sectioned into three parts and woven together (also referred to as *plaits.*) Can be styled with only the hair that grows out of one's head, or by adding hair extensions for length and/or easier maintenance.

CORNROWS *n.* Hair that is braided along the scalp by adding additional pieces of hair in a desired direction.

CREAMY CRACK *n.* A phrase referring to the chemicals used to relax hair. Relaxers have a thick, creamy like substance and like cocaine, are white. Implies that those who use relaxers have an obsessive, drug-like dependence on hair straightening.

GOOD HAIR *adj.* A term in Black culture used to describe hair that is naturally straighter in texture. *Good hair* usually means wavy or curly, but is not tightly coiled enough to be considered nappy or kinky. Defined as the opposite of *bad hair* or *nappy hair* and is perceived as more beautiful and manageable. Natural hair communities tend to redefine good hair as healthy hair of any texture in resistance to texturism.

HAIR TYPING *n.* Systems that classify hair into categories. The most popular hair typing system, popularized by celebrity stylist Andre Walker, classifies texture into four categories: 1 (straight), 2 (wavy), 3 (curly), and 4 (kinky or coily). Each category is further broken down into A, B, and C for more detail. Some believe that hair typing presents hair texture in a hierarchical manner and reinforces texturism and good/bad hair grades, while others find the system helps them describe their hair in more detail and find influencers to follow whose curl pattern is like their own. In addition to typing curl pattern, discussions in natural hair culture often but less frequently type hair by porosity, or the degree to which a person's hair absorbs and holds moisture, density, or how close strands are to one another, and the thickness of individual strands of hair.

INFLUENCER *n.* An individual who uses his or her popularity on social media networking sites or blogs to influence the opinions, behavior, taste, or consumer choices of his or her following. Being an influencer is a web 2.0 form of celebrity and entrepreneurship that relies on digital content creation, sponsorship from companies, and/or residuals from video views. For natural hair influencers, content creation often takes the form of reviewing and marketing hair products, creating styling tutorials, or writing opinion pieces about beauty culture. Natural hair influencers are highly sought after to make guest appearances at natural hair shows. Some create their own natural hair tour "meet and greets" to monetize authority offline.

LINE OF DEMARCATION *n.* The point where virgin and processed hair meet.

LOCS (*also referred to as dreadlocks, or dreads*), *n.* HAir that is matted together, or "locked," in rope-like sections. Has roots in the

Rastafarian religion, but many wear locs as a political statement, fashion choice, or for convenience. Some locs are grown freeform, where hair is left to group and create sections on its own. Others deliberately style locs by parting and twisting or braiding hair into even sections to start the locking process. *Sisterlocks* and *Brotherlocks* are an increasingly popular form of tiny locs originated by Dr. JoAnne Cornwell in 1993, where hair is sectioned into a small grid and knotted together using a specialized tool.

NAPPY *adj* A term for natural hair textures that are kinky or tightly coiled. Often used in a derogatory sense and defined as the negative opposite of *good hair*. However, many Black communities have reclaimed term as a celebratory or value-neutral descriptive term for tightly coiled hair.

NATURAL *adj.* 1) Hair that has not been processed by chemical relaxers and is worn in a state that does not require straightening of any kind. Dreadlocks are considered a natural hairstyle. Braids, cornrows, twists and twist-outs are also considered natural hairstyles even though they require manipulating hair and may result in mechanically altering hair texture. 2) In reference to products, natural refers to goods that are free from chemicals like preservatives, parabens, silicones, and sulfates.

PRODUCT JUNKIE *n.* A person who has amassed a large collection of natural hair products. Consumers tend to become product junkies if they enjoy trying out new items or because they have not yet learned what products work well for their hair texture, desired look, or lifestyle. An online culture in which influencers review natural hair products and a natural hair meet-up culture centered around vendors likely contributes to the product junkie phenomenon.

PROTECTIVE STYLE *n.* A style worn for multiple days, weeks, or months at a time in order to reduce the need to manipulate one's hair. Popular protective styles include two-strand twists, braids, and cornrows. Some women wear weaves and wigs as protective styles.

RELAXED HAIR (permed hair) *n.* Hair that has been permanently straightened by applying a chemical solution of sodium hydroxide (lye) or calcium hydroxide (no lye).

TEXTURISM *n.* A belief that straighter hair is more beautiful, feminine, and superior. In natural hair communities, texturism contributes to the overrepresentation of women with wavy and curly hair, and the underrepresentation of women with tightly coiled or kinky hair.

TRANSITIONING *v.* The process of growing out chemically-treated or damaged hair to reveal one's natural hair texture. Transitioning typically happens in one of two ways: 1) Big chopping by shaving the entire head at once or 2) growing out relaxed or damaged hair over time to retain a desired hair length.

TWA "TEENY WEENY AFRO" *n.* Short hair in beginning stages of transition, just after a "big chop."

TWO STRAND TWISTS *n.* A popular protective style for natural hair achieved by weaving two strands of hair around each other. A "twist out" is a hairstyle where two strand twists are unwoven after hair has had time take on the spiral texture from the twists. "Senegalese twists" are a hairstyle in which synthetic hair is added to small, twisted sections.

WASH DAY *n.* A day of the week set aside for self-care through hair care.

WEAVE *n.* A hairstyle in which wefts of synthetic or human hair are sewn, glued, or bonded over one's own plaited or cornrowed hair.

NOTES

INTRODUCTION

1 Collins, 2000, *Black Feminist Thought*; Crenshaw, 1991, "Mapping the Margins"; Collins, 1986, "Learning from the Outsider Within."
2 Weitz, 2005, *Rapunzel's Daughters*.
3 Mercer, 1994, *Welcome to the Jungle*, 103.
4 Wingfield, 2008, *Doing Business with Beauty*.
5 Omi and Winant, 1994, *Racial Formation in the United States*.
6 Candis Tate, 2016, "Loving Blackness," 1.
7 Cullors, 2018, *When They Call You a Terrorist*; Lebron, 2017, *Making of Black Lives Matter*; Ransby, 2018, *Making All Black Lives Matter*; Keeanga-Yamahtta Taylor, 2016, *From #BlackLivesMatter to Black Liberation*.
8 Bordo, 1993, *Unbearable Weight*.
9 Wingfield, 2008, *Doing Business with Beauty*; Collins, 2005, *Black Sexual Politics*; Nagel, 2003, *Race, Ethnicity, and Sexuality*.
10 Springer, 2007, "Divas, Evil Black Bitches, and Bitter Black Women"; Collins, 2000, *Black Feminist Thought*; Gilkes, 1983, "From Slavery to Social Welfare."
11 hooks, 2014, *Ain't I a Woman*; Collins, 2005, *Black Sexual Politics*; Hays, 2004, *Flat Broke with Children*
12 Weitz, 2009, "A History of Women's Bodies"; Nagel, 2003, *Race, Ethnicity, and Sexuality*; Collins, 2000, *Black Feminist Thought*; Gilkes, 1983, "From Slavery to Social Welfare."
13 Banks, 2000, *Hair Matters*; Rooks, 1996, *Hair Raising*.
14 Jha, 2015, *Global Beauty Industry*; Mears, 2011, *Pricing Beauty*; Craig, 2006, "Race, Beauty, and the Tangled Knot of a Guilty Pleasure"; Banks, 2000, *Hair Matters*; McCaughey, 1998, "The Fighting Spirit"; Rooks, 1996, *Hair Raising*.
15 Jha, 2015, *Global Beauty Industry*; Hunter, 2005, *Race, Gender, and the Politics of Skin Tone*.
16 Hochschild and Weaver, 2007, "Skin Color Paradox," 643.
17 See glossary for definitions of common natural hair terminology.
18 Thompson, 2009, "Black Women, Beauty, and Hair"; Hunter, 2005, *Race, Gender, and the Politics of Skin Tone*.
19 Jha, 2015, *Global Beauty Industry*; Elizabeth Johnson, *Resistance and Empowerment in Black Women's Hair Styling*; Mears, 2011, *Pricing Beauty*; Craig,

2002, *Ain't I a Beauty Queen?*; Collins, 2000, *Black Feminist Thought*; Banet-Weiser, *Most Beautiful Girl in the World*.

20 Mears, 2011, *Pricing Beauty*.

21 Jacobs-Huey, 2006, *From the Kitchen to the Parlor*, 3.

22 Byrd and Tharps, 2014, *Hair Story*; Rooks, 1996, *Hair Raising*; Mercer, 1994, *Welcome to the Jungle*.

23 Thompson, 2009, "Black Women, Beauty, and Hair."

24 Thompson, 2009, "Black Women, Beauty, and Hair"; Shirley Tate, 2007, "Black Beauty."

25 West and Zimmerman, 1987, "Doing Gender," 145.

26 Byrd and Tharps, 2014, *Hair Story*; Jacobs-Huey, 2006, *From the Kitchen to the Parlor*; Willett, 2000, *Permanent Waves*.

27 Banks, 2000, *Hair Matters*.

28 Thompson, 2009, "Black Women, Beauty, and Hair," 855.

29 McGill Johnson et al., 2017, "'Good Hair' Study." The Perception Institute surveyed a national sample of 4,163 participants using a computerized Implicit Association Test (IAT) that flashed images of Black women with textured or smooth hairstyles to document whether and how quickly participants associate pleasant words (like "love," "peace," and "happy") or unpleasant words (like "death," "hatred," "evil") with each image. Such tests have become common in social psychology since the mid-1990s and are designed to detect the strength of association between concepts and evaluations.

30 Koval and Rosette, 2021, "The Natural Hair Bias in Job Recruitment."

31 Banks, 2000, *Hair Matters*.

32 Collins, 2000, *Black Feminist Thought*, 82.

33 Adichie,2013, *Americanah*; Angela Davis, 1994, "Afro Images"; Toni Morrison, 1970, *Bluest Eye*; Robinson, 2016, *You Can't Touch My Hair*, Smith, 2000, *White Teeth*; Alice Walker, 1989, *Living by the Word*.

34 Wingfield, 2008, *Doing Business with Beauty*; Jacobs-Huey, 2006, *From the Kitchen to the Parlor*; Battle-Walters, 2004, *Sheila's Shop*; Mercer, 1994, *Welcome to the Jungle*.

35 Rowe, 2021, "Rooted"; Tinsley, 2018, *Beyoncé in Formation*.

36 Robinson, 2016, *You Can't Touch My Hair*, 6, original emphasis.

37 Balogun, 2012, "Cultural and Cosmopolitan"; Craig, 2002, *Ain't I a Beauty Queen?*

38 Balogun, 2012, "Cultural and Cosmopolitan"; King-O'Riain, 2006, *Pure Beauty*; Craig, 2002, *Ain't I a Beauty Queen?*; Banet-Weiser, 1999, *Most Beautiful Girl in the World*.

39 Bailey, 2010, "They Aren't Talking About Me."

40 I choose to use the term "movement" to reflect how natural hair communities have named their culture and described its meanings. This book would be illegible to those I interviewed and met in the field if I called the natural hair movement anything other than a movement, even if it does not meet every sociologist's criteria for one. I engage the sociological literature on social

movements to take seriously women's claims that natural hair has political implications. See also Saro-Wiwa's 2012 article for the *New York Times* on natural hair as a social movement. Saro-Wiwa, 2012, "Black Women's Transitions to Natural Hair."

41 Miles, 2018, "Black Hair's Blockbuster Moment."

42 I refer to my interviewees using pseudonyms throughout the text to protect their identities and confidentiality.

43 Falzon, 2009, *Multi-Sited Ethnography.*

44 Gilroy, 1993, *Black Atlantic.*

45 Ford, 2016, *Liberated Threads.*

46 Hallett and Barber, 2014, "Ethnographic Research in a Cyber Era."

47 Leslie McCall outlines three main approaches to intersectional research: 1) intercategorical, 2) anticategorical, and 3) intercategorical frameworks. The intercategorical approach, typically used by quantitative sociologists, strategically employs categories to measure and compare inequality *between* groups. The anticategorical approach to intersectionality evolves from postmodernist and poststructuralist critiques that cast suspicion on the validity of modern categories, and considers heterogeneity at the individual level too vast to grapple with difference within collectivities. While useful for analyzing individual experiences, anticategorical approaches often fail to acknowledge the lasting and meaningful affective relationships individuals have with larger identity-based communities. The intracategorical intersectional method employs identity categories even while remaining critical of them, focusing on a single intersection between multiple axes of identity. I take an intracategorical approach, recognizing that interlocking systems of power and privilege determine social location, and that people form solidarity by identifying with those who are similarly positioned. See McCall, 2005, "Complexity of Intersectionality."

1. HAIR SANKOFA

1 Green, 2012, *Rise of the Trans-Atlantic Slave Trade.*

2 Byrd and Tharps, 2014, *Hair Story.*

3 Green, 2012, *Rise of the Trans-Atlantic Slave Trade.*

4 Rawley and Behrendt, 2005, *Transatlantic Slave Trade.*

5 Omi and Winant, 1994, *Racial Formation in the United States*, 55.

6 Harris, 1993, "Whiteness as Property."

7 Cha-Jua, 2001, "Racial Formation and Transformation."

8 Omi and Winant, 1994, *Racial Formation in the United States.*

9 Byrd and Tharps, 2014, *Hair Story.*

10 Weitz, 2005, *Rapunzel's Daughters.*

11 Weitz, 2005, *Rapunzel's Daughters.*

12 Byrd and Tharps, 2014, *Hair Story.*

13 Work Projects Administration, 1936, *Federal Writers' Project*, 18.

14   Russell-Cole, Wilson, and Hall, 1993, *Color Complex*.

15   Mercer, 1994, *Welcome to the Jungle*, 101.

16   Byrd and Tharps, 2014, *Hair Story*, 174.

17   Jha, 2015, *Global Beauty Industry*; Russell-Cole, Wilson, and Cole, 1993, *Color Complex*; Glenn, 2008, "Yearning for Lightness"; Shirley Tate, 2007, "Black Beauty"; Hunter, 2005, *Race, Gender, and the Politics of Skin Tone*.

18   Angela Davis, 1981, *Women, Race, and Class*.

19   Russell-Cole, Wilson, and Hall, 1993, *Color Complex*; Angela Davis, 1981, *Women, Race, and Class*.

20   Byrd and Tharps, 2014, *Hair Story*.

21   Kandaswamy, 2012, "Gendering Racial Formation"; Ferguson, 2012, "On the Specificities of Racial Formation"; Kitch, 2009, *Specter of Sex*.

22   Collins, 2005, *Black Sexual Politics*.

23   Angela Davis, 1981, *Women, Race, and Class*.

24   Byrd and Tharps, 2014, *Hair Story*; Russell-Cole, Wilson, and Hall, 1993, *Color Complex*; Angela Davis, 1981, *Women, Race, and Class*.

25   Russell-Cole, Wilson, and Hall, 1993, *Color Complex*.

26   Weitz, 2005, *Rapunzel's Daughters*, 39.

27   Byrd and Tharps, 2014, *Hair Story*; Weitz, 2005, *Rapunzel's Daughters*.

28   Bell, 1997, *Revolution, Romanticism, and the Afro-Creole Protest Tradition*.

29   Lemire, 2018, *Global Trade and the Transformation of Consumer Cultures*.

30   Omi and Winant, 1994, *Racial Formation in the United States*, 327.

31   Marques, 2016, *United States and the Transatlantic Slave Trade*.

32   Lemire, 2018, *Global Trade and the Transformation of Consumer Cultures*, 112.

33   Lowe, 1996, *Immigrant Acts*.

34   Quoted in Byrd and Tharps, 2014, *Hair Story*, 74.

35   Willett, 2000, *Permanent Waves*.

36   Bristol, 2009, *Knights of the Razor*.

37   Wingfield, 2008, *Doing Business with Beauty*.

38   Blackwelder, 2003, *Styling Jim Crow*.

39   Bundles, 2001, "Madam C. J. Walker."

40   Juliet Walker, 2009, *History of Black Business in America*.

41   Byrd and Tharps, 2014, *Hair Story*.

42   Tiffany Gill, 2001, "'I Had My Own Business.'"

43   Tiffany Gill, 2001, "'I Had My Own Business.'"

44   Blackwelder, 2003, *Styling Jim Crow*.

45   Tiffany Gill, 2010, *Beauty Shop Politics*.

46   Tiffany Gill, 2010, *Beauty Shop Politics*; Blackwelder, 2003, *Styling Jim Crow*; Tiffany Gill, 2001, "'I Had My Own Business'"; Willett, 2000, *Permanent Waves*.

47   Tiffany Gill, *Beauty Shop Politics*.

48   Blackwelder, 2003, *Styling Jim Crow*.

49 Tiffany Gill, 2001, "'I Had My Own Business,'" 190.

50 Craig, 2002, *Ain't I a Beauty Queen?*; Bundles, 2001, "Madam C. J. Walker"; Tiffany Gill, 2001, "'I Had My Own Business'"; Susannah Walker, 2000, "Black is Profitable"; Rooks, 1996, *Hair Raising.*

51 Higginbotham, 1993, *Righteous Discontent.*

52 Collins, 2000, *Black Sexual Politics*; Craig, 2002, *Ain't I a Beauty Queen?*; Banks, 2000, *Hair Matters*; Higginbotham, 1993, *Righteous Discontent.*

53 Blackwelder, 2003, *Styling Jim Crow*, 6.

54 Elizabeth Johnson, 2013, *Resistance and Empowerment in Black Women's Hair*; Craig, 2006, "Race, Beauty, and the Tangled Knot of a Guilty Pleasure"; Mitchell, 2004, *Righteous Propagation*; Higginbotham, 1993, *Righteous Discontent.*

55 X and Haley, 1964, *Autobiography of Malcolm X*, 64.

56 X and Haley, 1964, *Autobiography of Malcolm X*, 64.

57 X and Haley, 1964, *Autobiography of Malcolm X*, 65.

58 Posel, 2001b, "What's in a Name?," 72.

59 Posel, 2001b, "What's in a Name?"

60 Byrd and Tharps, 2014, *Hair Story*; Russell-Cole, Wilson, and Hall, 1993, *Color Complex*; Craig, 2002, *Ain't I a Beauty Queen?*; Tiffany Gill, 2001, "'I Had My Own Business.'"

61 Byrd and Tharps, 2014, *Hair Story*; Lake, 2003, *Blue Veins and Kinky Hair*; Russell-Cole, Wilson, and Hall, 1993, *Color Complex.*

62 Craig, 2002, *Ain't I a Beauty Queen?*

63 Jacobs-Huey, 2006, *From the Kitchen to the Parlor*; Battle-Walters, 2004, *Sheila's Shop*; Banks, 2000, *Hair Matters*; Rooks, 1996, *Hair Raising.*

64 Kia Caldwell, 2007, *Negras in Brazil.*

65 Byrd and Tharps, 2014, *Hair Story*; Craig, 2006, "Race, Beauty, and the Tangled Knot of a Guilty Pleasure"; Craig, 2002, *Ain't I a Beauty Queen?*

66 Byrd and Tharps, 2014, *Hair Story.*

67 Du Bois, 1903, *Souls of Black Folk*, 9.

68 Stille, 2007, *Madam C. J. Walker*; Bundles, 2001, "Madam C. J. Walker"; Rooks, 1996, *Hair Raising.*

69 Craig, 2002, *Ain't I a Beauty Queen?*

70 Byrd and Tharps, 2014, *Hair Story.*

71 Willett, 2000, *Permanent Waves.*

72 Ture and Hamilton, 1992, *Black Power.*

73 Craig, 2002, *Ain't I a Beauty Queen?*, 18.

74 Mercer, 1994, *Welcome to the Jungle.*

75 Susannah Walker, 2000, "Black Is Profitable."

76 Byrd and Tharps, 2014, *Hair Story*; Walker, 2000, "Black Is Profitable."

77 Ford, 2016, *Liberated Threads*, 7.

78 Craig, 2006, "Race, Beauty, and the Tangled Knot of a Guilty Pleasure," 172.

79 Ford, 2016, *Liberated Threads*; Mercer, 1994, *Welcome to the Jungle*.

80 Craig, 2006, "Race, Beauty, and the Tangled Knot of a Guilty Pleasure"; Banks, 2000, *Hair Matters*; Mercer, 1994, *Welcome to the Jungle*.

81 Craig, 2006, "Race, Beauty, and the Tangled Knot of a Guilty Pleasure"; Angeline Morrison, 2006, "Black Skin, Big Hair"; Mercer, 1994, *Welcome to the Jungle*.

82 Angeline Morrison, 2006, "Black Skin, Big Hair," 106.

83 Mercer, 1994, *Welcome to the Jungle*; Ford, 2016, *Liberated Threads*.

84 Mercer, 1994, *Welcome to the Jungle*.

85 Ford, 2016, *Liberated Threads*.

86 Kelley, 1997, "Nap Time," 348.

87 Craig, 2006, "Race, Beauty, and the Tangled Knot of a Guilty Pleasure."

88 Angela Davis, 1994, "Afro Images," 42.

89 Byrd and Tharps, 2014, *Hair Story*; Ford, 2016, *Liberated Threads*; Banks, 2000, *Hair Matters*.

90 Mercer, 1994, *Welcome to the Jungle*.

91 Willett, 2000, *Permanent Waves*.

92 Walker, 2000; Davis, 1994.

93 Susannah Walker, 2007, *Style and Status*; Susannah Walker, 2000, "Black Is Profitable."

94 Angela Davis, 1994, "Afro Images," 37.

95 Byrd and Tharps, 2014, *Hair Story*; Willett, 2000, *Permanent Waves*.

96 Tiffany Gill, 2010, *Beauty Shop Politics*; McAndrew, 2010, "A Twentieth Century Triangle Trade."

97 McAndrew, 2010, "A Twentieth Century Triangle Trade," 798.

98 Tiffany Gill, 2010, *Beauty Shop Politics*.

99 Mears, 2011, *Pricing Beauty*.

100 Rose, 1994, *Black Noise*.

101 Lipsitz, 2006, *Possessive Investment in Whiteness*.

102 Timothy Brown, 2005, "Allen Iverson as America's Most Wanted," 78.

103 Mercer, 1994, *Welcome to the Jungle*.

104 Timothy Brown, 2005, "Allen Iverson as America's Most Wanted," 81.

105 Carbado and Harris, 2012, "New Racial Preferences"; Ansell, 2006, "Casting a Blind Eye"; Bonilla-Silva, *Racism Without Racists*.

106 Thompson, 2009, "Black Women, Beauty, and Hair"; Carbado and Harris, 2012, "New Racial Preferences"; Collins, 2005, *Black Sexual Politics*; Craig, 2002, *Ain't I a Beauty Queen?*; Banks, 2000, *Hair Matters*; Kia Caldwell, 2007, *Negras in Brazil*.

107 Collins, 1998, *Fighting Words*, 38.

108 Lorde, 1984, *Sister Outsider*, 288.

109 Carbado, 2013, "Colorblind Intersectionality"; Paulette Caldwell, 2008, "Intersectional Bias and the Courts"; Crenshaw, 1989, "Demarginalizing the Intersection of Race and Sex."

110 Byrd and Tharps, 2014, *Hair Story*.

111 Juliet Walker, 2009, *History of Black Business in America*, xvi.

112 Feagin and Elias, 2013, "Rethinking Racial Formation Theory"; Juliet Walker, 2009, *History of Black Business in America*; Lipsitz, 2006, *Possessive Investment in Whiteness*.

113 Byrd and Tharps, 2014, *Hair Story*.

114 Doherty, 1987, "Advertising: Essence Bans Ads of Revlon."

115 Wingfield, 2008, *Doing Business with Beauty*; Yoon, 2007, *On My Own*; Silverman, *Doing Business in Minority Markets*; Light and Bonacich, 1988, *Immigrant Entrepreneurs*.

116 Yoon, 2007, *On My Own*.

117 Yoon, 2007, *On My Own*; Portes and Jenson, 1989, "Enclave and the Entrants"; Bonacich, 1973, "A Theory of Middleman Minorities."

118 Byrd and Tharps, 2014, *Hair Story*.

119 Byrd and Tharps, 2014, *Hair Story*; Yoon, 2007, *On My Own*.

120 Lipsitz, 2006, *Possessive Investment in Whiteness*, 4.

121 Kim, 1993, "Racial Triangulation of Asian Americans."

122 Mears, 2011, *Pricing Beauty*, 5.

123 Elizabeth Johnson, 2013, *Resistance and Empowerment in Black Women's Hair Styling*.

124 Byrd and Tharps, 2014, *Hair Story*.

2. LIBERATING TRANSITIONS

1 Carr, 1997, *"Colorblind" Racism*.

2 Bonilla-Silva, 2006, *Racism Without Racists*.

3 Cooky, Wachs, Messner, and Dworkin, 2010, "It's Not About the Game."

4 Carbado, 2013, "Colorblind Intersectionality"; Paulette Caldwell, 1991, "Hair Piece."

5 Finley, 2016, "Appeals Court Rules Employers."

6 Salhotra, 2024, "Judge says Texas school district can punish Black student for length of his hairstyle."

7 Collins, 1998, *Fighting Words*, 38.

8 US General Accounting Office, 2000, "Better Targeting of Airline Passengers." The report's recommendations to use a data-driven approach to target passengers for search was not adopted by the TSA.

9 Browne, 2015, *Dark Matters*, 132.

10 Browne, 2015, *Dark Matters*, 29.

11 Mercer, 1994, *Welcome to the Jungle*.

12 American Civil Liberties Union of Northern California, 2015, "ACLU and TSA Reach Agreement."

13 Evans and Riley, 2013, "Immaculate Consumption," 271.

14 Psychiatrist Chester Pierce first coined the term microaggression in *Offensive Mechanisms* to describe common insults and dismissals based in racist

stereotypes that he observed non-Black Americans target toward Black Americans. Applying an intersectional approach, researchers have since used the term to describe slights against other marginalized social groups, including immigrants, members of the LGBTQ community, the disabled, and women of color. Health scientists have proposed that the stress caused by microaggressions may explain psychological and physical health disparities facing middle-class Black women, who are more likely to live and work in isolation within predominantly white environments. See Sue, 2010, *Microaggressions in Everyday Life* for an overview on microaggressions and Lewis et al., 2017, "Applying Intersectionality" for an intersectional analysis on the relationship between microaggressions and Black women's health outcomes.

15 Rowe, 2021, "Rooted."

16 Moore, 2006, "Lipstick or Timberlands?"

17 Lyle, Jones, and Drakes, 1999, "Beauty on the Borderland," 52.

18 Weitz, 2005, *Rapunzel's Daughters*; Lyle, Jones, and Drakes, "Beauty on the Borderland."

19 Weitz, 2005, *Rapunzel's Daughters*.

20 Fischer, "A Letter to Black Trans Women about Embracing Our Natural Hair."

21 Judith Butler, *Undoing Gender*; Collins, 2005, *Black Sexual Politics*.

22 Byrd and Tharps, 2014, *Hair Story*; Banks, 2000, *Hair Matters*.

23 Weitz, 2005, *Rapunzel's Daughters*, 12.

24 Byrd and Tharps, 2014, *Hair Story*; Jacobs-Huey, 2006, *From the Kitchen to the Parlor*; Weitz, 2005, *Rapunzel's Daughters*; Banks, 2000, *Hair Matters*; Rooks, 1996, *Hair Raising*.

25 Candis Tate, 2016, "Loving Blackness," 38.

26 hooks, 2015b, *Sisters of the Yam*, xi.

27 This interview was conducted in writing via email in order to overcome our language barrier, and participant responses were translated from Portuguese to English using an automated tool.

28 Twine, 1998, *Racism in a Racial Democracy*.

29 Hordge-Freeman, 2015, *Color of Love*.

30 Bordo, 1993, *Unbearable Weight*; Wolf, 1991, *Beauty Myth*.

31 As of the time of publication, *Hair Nah* by Momo Pixel can still be played online at www.hairnah.com.

32 See glossary at the end of this book.

33 Tiffany Gill, 2015, "#TeamNatural."

34 McGill Johnson et al., 2017, "'Good Hair' Study."

35 Woolford et al., 2016, "No Sweat," 14.

36 Elizabeth Johnson, 2013, *Resistance and Empowerment in Black Women's Hair Styling*.

37 Ellington, 2014, "Social Networking Sites."

3. GREEN IS THE NEW BLACK

1 Hofman and Tugendhaft, 2016, "South Africans have a Sweet Tooth."

2 Black Women for Wellness, 2016, *Natural Evolutions*; Chang et al., 2022, "Use of Straighteners and other Hair Products and Incident Uterine Cancer"; Rosenberg et al., 2007, "Hair Relaxers not Associated with Breast Cancer."

3 Gibson-Wood and Wakefield, 2013, "Participation"; Mann, 2011, "Pioneers of U.S. Ecofeminism."

4 Gibson-Wood and Wakefield, 2013, "Participation"; Mann, 2011, "Pioneers of U.S. Ecofeminism"; Dorceta Taylor, 1997, "Women of Color, Environmental Justice, and Ecofeminism."

5 Quoted in Melosi, 2006, "Environmental Justice, Ecoracism, and Environmental History," 125.

6 Gaard, 2010, "Ecofeminism and Native American Cultures."

7 Mackendrick, 2014, "More Work for Mother"; Cairns, Johnston, and Mackendrick, 2013, "Feeding the 'Organic Child.'"

8 Sturgeon, 1997, *Ecofeminist Natures*.

9 Carbado, 2013, "Colorblind Intersectionality," 822.

10 Stiel et al., 2016, "A Review of Hair Product Use"; Black Women for Wellness, 2016, *Natural Evolutions*; Donovan et al., 2007, "Personal Care Products."

11 Rosenberg et al., 2007, "Hair Relaxers not Associated with Breast Cancer."

12 Donovan et al., 2007, "Personal Care Products."

13 Food and Drug Administration, 2022, "Cosmetic Labeling Guide."

14 Epstein and Fitzgerald, 2009, *Toxic Beauty*.

15 Donovan et al., 2007, "Personal Care Products"

16 Black Women for Wellness, 2016, *Natural Evolutions*; Wise et al., 2012, "Hair Relaxer Use."

17 Stiel et al., 2016, "A Review of Hair Product Use."

18 Wise et al., 2012, "Hair Relaxer Use."

19 Chang et al., 2022, "Use of Straighteners and other Hair Products and Incident Uterine Cancer."

20 Wise et al., 2012, "Hair Relaxer Use."

21 Tiffany Gill, 2015, "#TeamNatural"; Tiffany Gill, 2010, *Beauty Shop Politics*; Wingfield, 2008, *Doing Business with Beauty*; Jacobs-Huey, 2006, *From the Kitchen to the Parlor*.

22 Black Women for Wellness, 2016, *Natural Evolutions*; Donovan et al., 2007, "Personal Care Products"; Tiwary, 1998, "Premature Sexual Development."

23 Donovan et al., 2007, "Personal Care Products."

24 Black Women for Wellness, 2016, *Natural Evolutions*.

25 Food and Drug Administration, 2022, "Cosmetic Labeling Guide."

26 Wise et al., 2012, "Hair Relaxer Use."

27 James-Todd et al., 2011, "Childhood Hair Product Use."

28 Tiwary, 1998, "Premature Sexual Development."

29 Collins, 2000, *Black Feminist Thought*, 67.

30 Woolford et al., 2016, "No Sweat."

31 O'Connor, 2011, "Surgeon General Calls for Health Over Hair."

32 US Department of Health and Human Services Office of Minority Health, 2017, "Profile: Black/African Americans."

33 Centers for Disease Control and Prevention, 2014, *National Diabetes Statistics Report*.

34 Stilson, 2009, *Chris Rock's Good Hair*.

35 Tiffany Gill, 2015, "#TeamNatural."

36 Tiffany Gill, 2015, "#TeamNatural," 76.

37 Saro-Wiwa, 2012, "Black Women's Transitions to Natural Hair."

38 Collins, 1986, "Learning from the Outsider Within."

39 Saro-Wiwa, 2012, "Black Women's Transitions to Natural Hair."

40 Lorde, 1988, *A Burst of Light*, 130.

41 Zola, 1972, "Medicine as an Institution of Social Control."

42 Merianos, Vidurek, and King, 2013, "Medicalization of Female Beauty"; Bordo, 1993, *Unbearable Weight*; Haiken, 2000, "Making of the Modern Face"; Kaw, 1993, "Medicalization of Racial Features."

43 Duggan, 2003, *Twilight of Equality?*

44 Evans and Riley, 2013, "Immaculate Consumption"; Wolf, 1991, *Beauty Myth*.

45 Berkowitz, 2017, *Botox Nation*.

46 Kaw, 1993, "Medicalization of Racial Features."

47 Kauer, 2016, "Yoga Culture."

48 Byrd and Tharps, 2014, *Hair Story*, 212.

49 Mackendrick, 2014, "More Work for Mother."

50 "Coloured" is a term describing a multiracial ethnic group in South Africa, including people with Khoisan, Bantu, European, East Asian, and Southeast Asian ancestry. Given the combination of ethnicities, individuals and people within a family may have a variety of different hair textures, facial features, and skin tones ranging from very light to very deep. During apartheid, the South African government socially and spatially segregated the Coloured population from Black, Indian, and white communities, giving rise to a unique and vibrant Coloured culture.

51 Gottleib quoted in Melosi, 2006, "Environmental Justice, Ecoracism, and Environmental History," 123.

52 hooks, 2014, *Ain't I a Woman*; Mann, 2011, "Pioneers of U.S. Ecofeminism"; Roth, 2004, *Separate Roads to Feminism*; Dorceta Taylor, 1997, "Women of Color, Environmental Justice, and Ecofeminism"; Collins, 1986, "Learning from the Outsider Within"; Zinn, Cannon, Higgenbotham, and Thornton Dill, 1986, "Costs of Exclusionary Practices in Women's Studies."

53 Combahee River Collective, 1977, "A Black Feminist Statement"; hooks, 2014, Ain't I a Woman?

54 Roth, 2004, *Separate Roads to Feminism*; Collins, 1986, "Learning from the Outsider Within"; Zinn, Cannon, Higgenbotham and Thornton Dill, 1986, "Costs of Exclusionary Practices in Women's Studies."

55 Riley, 2004, "Ecology Is a Sistah's Issue Too," 414.

56 Riley, 2004, "Ecology Is a Sistah's Issue Too"; Plumwood, 1993, *Feminism and the Mastery of Nature*.

57 hooks and West, 1991, *Breaking Bread*, 153.

58 Garland-Thomson, 1996, "Cultural Work of American Freak Shows," 71.

59 Crais and Scully, 2009, *Sara Baartman*, 3.

60 Crais and Scully, 2009, *Sara Baartman*, 80.

61 Collins, 2005, *Black Sexual Politics*; Nagel, 2003, *Race, Ethnicity, and Sexuality*.

62 hooks and West, 1991, *Breaking Bread*; Collins, 2005, *Black Sexual Politics*.

63 Dorothy Roberts, 2016, *Killing the Black Body*; hooks and West, 1991, *Breaking Bread*; Collins, 2005, *Black Sexual Politics*.

64 Hancock, 2004, *Politics of Disgust*.

65 Dorothy Roberts, 2016, *Killing the Black Body*.

66 Heller, 2010, "For the Love of Nature," 230.

67 Collins, 2005, *Black Sexual Politics*.

68 Riley, 2004, "Ecology Is a Sistah's Issue Too," 414.

69 Berkowitz, 2017, *Botox Nation*; Kauer, 2016, "Yoga Culture."

70 Jess Butler, 2013, "For White Girls Only?," 41.

71 Gill and Scharff, 2011, *New Femininities*, 7.

72 Dworkin and Wachs, 2009, *Body Panic*.

73 Jess Butler, 2013, "For White Girls Only?"; McRobbie, 2009, *Aftermath of Feminism*; Rosalind Gill, *Gender and the Media*.

74 Jess Butler, 2013, "For White Girls Only?"; Gill and Scharff, 2011, *New Femininities*; McRobbie, 2009, *Aftermath of Feminism*; Duggan, 2003, *Twilight of Equality?*

75 Bordo, 1993, *Unbearable Weight*; Wolf, 1991, *Beauty Myth*; Bartky, 1990, *Femininity and Domination*.

76 Wolf, 1991, *Beauty Myth*.

77 Faludi, 2009, *Backlash*.

78 Elias, Gill, and Scharff, eds., 2017, *Aesthetic Labor*.

79 Wingfield, 2008, *Doing Business with Beauty*. The market research firm Mintel estimates that the Black haircare market will reach $761 million by 2017, and as much as half a trillion dollars if e-commerce, distributors, weaves, and independent beauty supply stores are considered in calculations. Tanya Roberts, 2014, "5 Trends Set to Shape the Black Haircare Market."

80 Elias, Gill, and Scarff, 2017, *Aesthetic Labor*; Jha, 2015, *Global Beauty Industry*; Craig, 2002, *Ain't I a Beauty Queen?*

81 Connell, 2009, *Gender*, 56.

82 Haug, 1987, *Female Sexualization*.

83 Wingfield, 2008, *Doing Business with Beauty*.

4. BLACK HAIR MATTERS

1 US Democratic Town Hall, February 23, 2016. Columbia, South Carolina.

2 De Lucca, 1999, "Unruly Arguments."

3 Peterson, 2011, "Militant Body and Political Communication."

4 Singer Beyoncé Knowles Carter was the headlining act for the 2016 Superbowl halftime show in Santa Clara, California, where she performed her hit single "Formation." The song was overtly political in nature, referencing the Black Lives Matter movement and the government's failure to protect Black New Orleanians after Hurricane Katrina in 2005. Costumed in black studded leather, flanked by background dancers in black berets staggered in an X formation, Beyoncé's styling and choreography nodded to the Black Panther Party's iconic uniform of rebellion, as well as to activist Malcom X. Beyoncé's performance was subsequently critiqued by right-wing politicians and catalyzed a protest at the NFL headquarters in New York City.

5 Michael Brown, an eighteen-year-old Black man, was fatally shot by Darren Wilson, a white police officer, in his hometown of Ferguson, Missouri, on August 9, 2014. Brown was accompanied by his friend Dorian Johnson, who reported that Brown held up his hands in surrender saying "don't shoot" after they both attempted to flee. The US Department of Justice ultimately concluded that Wilson shot Brown in self-defense. The killing and the ultimate failure to indict Wilson ignited many nights of protest and unrest in Ferguson, and remains a high-profile example of racialized police violence against Black men with impunity.

6 Sasson-Levy and Rapoport, 2003, "Body, Gender, and Knowledge."

7 Douglass, 1868 quoted in Chesebrough, 1998, *Frederick Douglass*, 67.

8 Truth, 1867, "When Woman Gets Her Rights," 38.

9 hooks, *Ain't I a Woman*; Collins, 1986, "Learning from the Outsider Within." Both texts describe the conflict between loving relationships with Black men and the desire for liberation from patriarchal oppression.

10 Wallace, 1990, *Black Macho*. The author uses her experience in the Black Panther Party to discuss the masculine biases and patriarchal culture of Black Power, despite its liberatory anti-racist agenda.

11 Roth, 2004, *Separate Roads to Feminism*; Wallace, 1990, *Black Macho*; Collins, 1986, "Learning from the Outsider Within."

12 Lorde, 1984, *Sister Outsider*, 291.

13 International Decolonial Black Feminism Summer School, Cachoiera, Bahia, Brazil, July 2017.

14 Craig, 2006, "Race, Beauty, and the Tangled Knot of a Guilty Pleasure"; Kelley, 1997, "Nap Time."

15 Lorde, 1984, *Sister Outsider*.

16 Rowe, 2021, "Rooted."

17 Roth, 2004, *Separate Roads to Feminism*; Laslett and Thorne, 1997, *Feminist Sociology*; hooks, 2014, *Ain't I a Woman*; Moraga and Anzaldúa, 1983, *This Bridge Called My Back*.

18 Angela Davis, 1981, *Women, Race, and Class.*

19 hooks, 2014, *Ain't I a Woman.*

20 McIntosh, 1989, "White Privilege."

21 Roth, 2004, *Separate Roads to Feminism.*

22 As Roth notes in *Separate Roads to Feminism (2004)*, the 1970s saw a rise in women of color organizing as a reaction to white-centered feminist organizing and experiences of sexism in nationalist and anti-racist organizing. Hijas de Cuauhtémoc and Comisión Femenil Mexicana Nacional are Chicana feminist organizations founded in 1971 and 1970, respectively. The Organization of Pan Asian American Women is a public policy organization founded in 1976 to address the concerns of Asian American women. The Combahee River Collective and the National Black Feminist Organization are organizations founded by African American women in 1974 and 1973, respectively, to address the unique issues facing Black women at the intersection of race, class, gender, and sexual oppression.

23 Walker, 1983, *In Search of Our Mothers' Gardens*, xi.

24 Lorde, 1984, *Sister Outsider.*

25 Combahee River Collective, 1977, "A Black Feminist Statement."

26 Zinn, Cannon, Higginbotham, and Thornton Dill, 1986, "Costs of Exclusionary Practices."

27 Collins, 2000, *Black Feminist Thought.*

28 Crenshaw, 1991, "Mapping the Margins"; Crenshaw, 1989, "Demarginalizing the Intersection of Race and Sex."

29 See Guy-Sheftall's *Words of Fire* for an excellent collection of Black feminist thought, including writing from early Black feminists such as Sojourner Truth and Anna Julia Cooper, who were theorizing their unique experiences at the intersection of racism, sexism, and class oppression as early as the mid-1800s. Guy-Sheftall, ed., 1995, *Words of Fire.*

30 Crenshaw et al., 2015, "Say Her Name," 4.

31 Brown et al., 2017, "#SayHerName."

32 Hull, Bell-Scott, and Smith, 1982, *All the Women are White.*

33 Chatelain and Asoka, 2015, "Women and Black Lives Matter," 56.

34 Ebonee Davis, 2016, "Black Girl Magic."

35 Krudy, 2016, "Justice Department Opens Criminal Probe."

36 Ebonee Davis, 2016, "Calvin Klein Model."

37 Ebonee Davis, 2016, "Calvin Klein Model."

38 Frank, 2017, "Eleventh Circuit Dreadlocks Ban." The 3–0 court decision ruled in favor of a Catastrophe Management Solutions's right to ask its employee, a Black woman named Chastity Jones, to cut her loc'ed hair to comply with the company's grooming policy. The EEOC relied on an argument that hairstyle can be changed and adopted by people of various racial backgrounds, thus does not meet the standard of an immutable characteristic of race or a feature subject to racial discrimination protections.

39 McGill Johnson et al., 2017, "'Good Hair' Study."

40 Saint Heron, 2016, "A Seat with Us."

41 Opiah, 2013, "You Can Touch My Hair."

42 Garland-Thomson, 1996, "Cultural Work of American Freak Shows."

43 Yancey, 2016, *Black Bodies, White Gazes*, xiii.

44 Baines, 1998, "Rainbow Nation?"

45 African National Congress, 1955, "Freedom Charter."

46 Anciano, 2014, "Non-Racialism in the African National Congress."

47 "Born free" refers to the generation born around the time of the first full and free democratic election in 1994.

48 Cecil John Rhodes was a British mining magnate and politician who served as Prime Minister for the Cape Colony, now South African, Zambia, and Zimbabwe, from 1890 to 1896. He is considered an early architect of apartheid because of his role in limiting the amount of land that Black Southern Africans were allowed to legally settle and his views on Anglo-British supremacy.

49 Biko, 1978, *Black Consciousness in South Africa*, 24.

50 The Soweto Uprisings were a series of youth-led demonstrations beginning the morning of June 16, 1976, in response to the introduction of Afrikaans language instruction in Black schools. Since the apartheid government was primarily run by white Afrikaners, the mandate was taken as an act of further oppression. By some estimates, as many as 20,000 students participated and as many as 700 students were killed by police. In honor and remembrance of the students' bravery, activism, and lives lost, June 16 is now a public holiday in South Africa, named "Youth Day."

51 Azania is an ancient name for Southern Africa used by indigenous Black groups and revived in recent times by several African nationalist organizations.

52 Sebambo, 2016, "Azania House as a Symbol of the Black Imagination," 108.

53 hooks, 2014, *Ain't I a Woman*.

54 Victor and Segun, 2016, "FeesMustFall."

55 Victor and Segun, 2016, "FeesMustFall," 7189.

56 Young, 1980, "Throwing Like a Girl."

57 For examples, see "'Racist School Hair Rules,'" *BBC News*, 2016; Mahr, 2016, "Protests over Black Girls' Hair"; Chigumadzi, 2016, "White Schools vs. Black Hair"; Chelsea Johnson, 2016, "Kinky, Curly Hair."

58 Samanga, 2017, "Why Racist Policies in South African Schools"; Parker, "Short Back and Sides."

59 ANC Women's League, 2016, "ANCWL Statement"; Democratic Alliance, 2016, "Outdated Gauteng School Policies."

60 Meyer and Whittier, 1994, "Social Movement Spillover."

61 Chigumadzi, 2016, "White Schools vs. Black Hair"; Nicholson, 2016, "South African Students Speak Out"; Mahr, 2016, "Protests over Black Girls' Hair"; BBC News, 2016, "'Racist School Hair Rules.'"

62 Collins and Bilge, 2016, *Intersectionality.*
63 Sutton, 2010, *Bodies in Crisis.*

5. WHO CAN BE NATURAL?

 1 McLaughlin and De Graaf, 2017, "So THAT'S How She Does It."
 2 Mercer, 1994, *Welcome to the Jungle.*
 3 Sunderland, 2015, "In Rachel Dolezal's Skin."
 4 Kara Brown, 2015, "Rachel Dolezal Definitely Nailed the Hair."
 5 Bensley, 2015, "How Rachel Dolezal Just Made Things Harder"; Warren, 2015, "Rachel Dolezal and Race as a Social Construct"; Luders-Manuel, 2015, "Mixed-Race Community's Response."
 6 Pichardo, 1997, "New Social Movements"; Buechler, 1995, "New Social Movement Theories."
 7 Polletta and Jasper, 2001, "Collective Identity and Social Movements"; Taylor and Whittier, 1999, "Collective Identity in Social Movement Communities."
 8 Taylor and Whittier, 1999, "Collective Identity in Social Movement Communities"; Rupp and Taylor, 1999, "Forging Feminist Identity."
 9 Taylor and Whittier, 1999, "Collective Identity in Social Movement Communities," 176.
10 Taylor and Whittier, 1999, "Collective Identity in Social Movement Communities," 174.
11 Carbado and Harris, 2012, "New Racial Preferences."
12 Lau, 2011, "New Bodies of Knowledge"; Roth, 2004, *Separate Roads to Feminism*; Crenshaw, 1991, "Mapping the Margins"; Combahee River Collective, 1977, "A Black Feminist Statement."
13 Formerly Julia Sudbury, the name under which her work appears in this book's reference list.
14 Sudbury, 2010, "(Re)constructing Multiracial Blackness."
15 Cooper, 2017, "SlutWalks vs. Ho Strolls," 48.
16 Craig, 2002, *Ain't I a Beauty Queen?*; Banks, 2000, *Hair Matters*; Mercer, 1994, *Welcome to the Jungle.*
17 Brubaker, 2016, "Dolezal Affair."
18 Young and Brunk, 2009, *Ethics of Cultural Appropriation*, 3.
19 Ko, 2014, "Can White Women be a Part of the Natural Hair Space?"
20 One noteworthy exception to a primary focus on white appropriation of Black cultural aesthetics is Nora Lum, a Chinese and Korean actress who has been criticized for her use of African American Vernacular English and use of the moniker Awkwafina, which some take to be inspired by African American names. Ma, 2021, "Negotiating Chineseness"; Makalintal, 2020, "Awkwafina's Past."
21 Angela Davis, 1994, "Afro Images," 37.
22 Pergament, 2015, "(Yes, You) Can Have an Afro.*"

23 Sherronda Brown, 2019, "Unruly: Subverting Body Terrorism by Celebrating Black Hair."

24 The term "blackfishing" is a play on the term "catfishing," a colloquialism to describe faking or impersonating someone online. Blackfishing refers to the practice of (mostly) white women using makeup, hairstyle, and fashion originating in Black culture to gain popularity on the internet, which can be leveraged for material gain through sponsorships and advertising deals. Cherid, 2021, "'Ain't Got Enough Money to Pay Me Respect'"; Stevens, 2021, "Blackfishing on Instagram"; Shirley Tate, 2021, "'I Do Not See Myself as Anything Else than White': Black Resistance to Racial Cosplay Blackfishing."

25 Aktar, 2016, "UFC Is Inspiring the Hottest New Hair Trend."

26 Paulette Caldwell, 1991, "Hair Piece."

27 Kara Brown, 2016, "White People Are Rebranding Cornrows as Boxer Braids."

28 E. Patrick Johnson, 2003, *Appropriating Blackness*, 5.

29 hooks, 2015b, *Black Looks*, 23.

30 Collins, 2005, *Black Sexual Politics*; Craig, 2002, *Ain't I a Beauty Queen?*; Banks, 2000, *Hair Matters*; Angela Davis, 1994, "Afro Images"; Paulette Caldwell, 1991, "Hair Piece."

31 quoted in Fuller, 2015, "Teen Vogue Slammed."

32 E. Patrick Johnson, 2003, *Appropriating Blackness*, 3.

33 L'Oréal, 2014, "L'Oréal USA Signs Agreement."

34 Patrice, 2014, "Beauty Conglomerate L'Oréal."

35 Ng and Dezember, 2015, "Bain Capital to Take Minority Stake."

36 Sundial Brands, 2015, "10 Reasons We Chose a New Partner."

37 Jerkins, 2017, "Whitewashing of Natural Hair Care Lines."

38 SheaMoisture, 2017 on Facebook. Quoted in Callahan, 2017, "Black Women are Upset over SheaMoisture."

39 Nielsen Company, 2017, "African American Women," 2.

40 "Black Twitter" is a term for the vibrant, informal virtual community, largely consisting of African American Twitter users, which shares a language, communication style, digital space, and collective voice online. It has become a space for cultural commentary, critique, humor, and protest. Many social movements have been conceived of or amplified by Black Twitter, as evidenced by hashtags like #BlackLivesMatter, which calls attention to state violence against African Americans, #OscarsSoWhite, which critiqued the lack of diversity at the Academy Awards and representation in Hollywood, and #BlackGirlMagic, which praises the accomplishments of Black women and girls; each have extended beyond the digital walls of Twitter to inspire change in organizations, schools, and traditional media.

41 Foster (@KimberlyNFoster), 2017.

42 SheaMoisture (@Sheamoisture), 2017.

43 Black Lives Matter, 2017, "Herstory."

44 Carney, 2016, "All Lives Matter, but So Does Race."

45 Yancey and Butler, 2015, "What's Wrong With 'All Lives Matter'?"

46 Sudbury, 2010, "(Re)constructing Multiracial Blackness," 36.

47 Ford, 2016, *Liberated Threads*; Byrd and Tharps, 2014, *Hair Story*; Mercer, 1994, *Welcome to the Jungle*.

48 Bonilla-Silva, 2006, *Racism Without Racists*; Carr, 1997, *"Colorblind" Racism*.

49 See Appendix A for reflections on race, embodiment, and the research process.

50 Jha, 2015, *Global Beauty Industry*.

51 Rowe, 2021, "Beyond 'Becky with the Good Hair.'"

52 White, 2024, "Beyoncé, The Boss."

53 See glossary entry for "Hair Typing."

54 Craig, 2002, *Ain't I a Beauty Queen?*

55 Duke, 2015, *Light Girls*.

56 Howze, 2017, "Free Yo Edges," 121.

57 Howze, 2017, "Free Yo Edges," 121.

58 Blay, 2016, "Let's Talk about Colorism."

59 Guy (@Auset_ntru, 2016).

60 Brown's article was originally published on the website Roaring Gold in 2017. The site was shut down by the owner and all content has been lost.

61 Posel, 2001a, "Race as Common Sense."

62 Oluo, 2017, "Heart of Whiteness."

63 Omi and Winant, 1994, *Racial Formation in the United States*.

64 Collins, 2000, *Black Feminist Thought*.

CONCLUSION

1 Jess Butler, 2013, "For White Girls Only?"; Gill and Scharff, 2011, *New Femininities*; McRobbie, 2009, *Aftermath of Feminism*; Rosalind Gill, 2007, *Gender and the Media*; Duggan, 2003, *Twilight of Equality?*

2 Black Women for Wellness, 2016, *Natural Evolutions*; Stiel et al., 2016, "A Review of Hair Product Use"; Wise et al., 2012, "Hair Relaxer Use"; Donovan et al., 2007, "Personal Care Products"; Rosenberg et al., 2007, "Hair Relaxers Not Associated with Breast Cancer Risk."

3 Bristol, 2009, *Knights of the Razor*.

4 Barber, 2016, *Styling Masculinity*.

5 Lorde, 1984, *Sister Outsider*.

6 Salhotra, 2024, "Judge says Texas school district can punish Black student for length of his hairstyle."

7 Bailey, 2010, "They Aren't Talking About Me."

APPENDIX A

1 Berg, 2001, *Qualitative Research Methods*.

2 Chelsea Johnson, 2017, "Bossiekop Is Beautiful"; Chelsea Johnson, 2016, "Black Beauty and the Economics of Liberation"; Chelsea Johnson, 2018, "10 Books by

Academics"; Chelsea Johnson, 2017, "What Your Hair Really Says About You"; Chelsea Johnson, 2017, "How Beauty Myths Are Holding Women Back Today"; Chelsea Johnson, 2018, "History of Headwraps"; Chelsea Johnson, "What It's Like Having Natural Hair in South Africa: #CurlsAroundtheWorld"; Chelsea Johnson, 2016, "My Natural, My Politics, My Way"; Chelsea Johnson, 2016, "Kinky, Curly Hair."

3 Jacobs-Huey, 2006, *From the Kitchen to the Parlor.*

4 Mears, 2011, *Pricing Beauty*; Kang, *Managed Hand*; Jacobs-Huey, 2006, *From the Kitchen to the Parlor*; Banks, 2000, *Hair Matters*; Weitz, 2005, *Rapunzel's Daughters.*

5 Mears, 2011, *Pricing Beauty.*

REFERENCES

Adichie, Chimamanda Ngozi. 2013. *Americanah*. New York: Alfred A. Knopf.

African National Congress. 1955. "Freedom Charter." Accessed February 9, 2018. https://www.anc1912.org.za/the-freedom-charter-2/.

Aktar, Alev. 2016. "UFC is Inspiring the Hottest New Hair Trend." *New York Post*. March 14, 2016. www.nypost.com.

American Civil Liberties Union of Northern California. 2015. "ACLU and TSA Reach Agreement over Racial Profiling of Black Women's Hair." March 26, 2015. www.aclunc.org.

ANC Women's League. 2016. "The ANCWL Statement on Racist Attacks on Learners at the Pretoria Girls High School by the School Management and their Rented Bouncers." Politics Web. August 29, 2016. Accessed September 1, 2016. https://www.politicsweb.co.za/politics/pghs-south-africans-should-not-tolerate-any-form-0.

Anciano, Fiona. 2014. "Non-Racialism in the African National Congress: Views from the Branch." *Journal of Contemporary African Studies* 32 (1): 35–55.

Ansell, Amy. 2006. "Casting a Blind Eye: The Ironic Consequences of Color-Blindness in South Africa and the United States." *Critical Sociology* 32 (2–3): 333–356.

Arie, India, Shannon Sanders, and Drew Ramsey. 2006. "I Am Not My Hair." *Testimony: Vol. 1, Life and Relationship*. Motown Records.

Bailey, Moya. 2010. "They Aren't Talking About Me." *Crunk Feminist Collective*. March 14, 2010. www.crunkfeministcollective.com.

Baines, Gary. 1998. "The Rainbow Nation? Identity and Nation Building in Post-Apartheid South Africa." *Mots Pluriels* 7:1–12.

Balogun, Oluwakemi. 2012. "Cultural and Cosmopolitan." *Gender & Society* 26 (3): 357–381.

Banet-Weiser, Sarah. 1999. *The Most Beautiful Girl in the World: Beauty Pageants and National Identity*. Berkeley: University of California Press.

Banks, Ingrid. 2000. *Hair Matters: Beauty, Power, and Black Women's Consciousness*. New York: New York University Press.

Barber, Kristen. 2016. *Styling Masculinity: Gender, Class, and Inequality in the Men's Grooming Industry*. New Brunswick, NJ: Rutgers University Press.

Bartky, Sandra Lee. 1990. *Femininity and Domination: Studies in the Phenomenology of Oppression*. New York: Routledge.

Battle-Walters, Kimberly. 2004. *Sheila's Shop: Working-Class African American Women Talk about Life, Love, Race and Hair*. Lanham, MD: Rowman and Littlefield.

Bell, Caryn Cossé. 1997. *Revolution, Romanticism, and the Afro-Creole Protest Tradition in Louisiana, 1718–1868*. Baton Rouge: Louisiana State University Press.

Bensley, Lisa. 2015. "How Rachel Dolezal Just Made Things Harder for Those of Us Who Don't 'Look Black.'" Black Girl with Long Hair. June 22, 2015. www.bglh-marketplace .com.

Berg, Bruce. 2001. *Qualitative Research Methods for the Social Sciences*. Boston: Allyn and Bacon.

Berkowitz, Dana. 2017. *Botox Nation: Changing the Face of America*. New York: New York University Press.

Biko, Steve. 1978. *Black Consciousness in South Africa*. New York: Vintage Books.

Black Lives Matter. 2017. "Herstory." Accessed February 28, 2024. www.Blacklivesmatter .com/about/herstory/.

Black Women for Wellness. 2016. *Natural Evolutions: One Hair Story*. Accessed January 1, 2021. www.bwwla.org.

Blackwelder, Julia. 2003. *Styling Jim Crow: African American Beauty Training During Segregation*. College Station: Texas A&M University Press.

Blay, Zeba. 2016. "Let's Talk about Colorism in the Natural Hair Community." *Huffington Post*. January 5, 2016. www.huffingtonpost.com.

Bonacich, Edna. 1973. "A Theory of Middleman Minorities." *American Sociological Review*, 38 (5): 583–594.

Bonilla-Silva, Eduardo. 2006. *Racism Without Racists: Colorblind Racism and the Persistence of Racial Inequality in America*. New York: Rowman & Littlefield.

Bordo, Susan. 1993. *Unbearable Weight: Feminism, Western Culture, and the Body*. Berkeley: University of California Press.

Bristol, Douglas W. 2009. *Knights of the Razor: Black Barbers in Slavery and Freedom*. Baltimore: Johns Hopkins University Press.

Brown, Kara. 2015. "Rachel Dolezal Definitely Nailed the Hair, I'll Give Her That." *Jezebel*. June 12, 2015. Accessed February 28, 2024. www.jezebel.com.

———. 2016. "White People Are Rebranding Cornrows as 'Boxer Braids.'" Jezebel. March 15, 2016. www.jezebel.com.

Brown, Melissa, Rashawn Ray, Ed Summers, and Neil Fraistat. 2017. "#SayHerName: A Case Study of Intersectional Social Media Activism." *Ethnic and Racial Studies* 40 (11): 1831–1846.

Brown, Sherronda. 2019. "Unruly: Subverting Body Terrorism by Celebrating Black Hair." *Wear Your Voice Mag*. February 11, 2019. Accessed December 28, 2021. www .wearyourvoicemag.com.

Brown, Timothy J. 2005. "Allen Iverson as America's Most Wanted: Black Masculinity as a Cultural Site of Struggle." *Journal of Intercultural Communications Research* 34 (1): 65–87.

Browne, Simone. 2015. *Dark Matters: On the Surveillance of Blackness*. Durham, NC: Duke University Press.

Brubaker, Rogers. 2016. "The Dolezal Affair: Race, Gender and the Micropolitics of Identity." *Ethnic and Racial Studies* 39 (3): 414–448.

Buechler. Steven M. 1995. "New Social Movement Theories." *The Sociological Quarterly* 36 (3): 441–464.

Bundles, A'lelia. 2001. "Madam C. J. Walker: 'Let Me Correct the Erroneous Impression that I Claim to Straighten Hair.'" In *Tenderheaded: A Comb-Bending Collection of Hair Stories*, edited by Juliette Harris and Pamela Johnson, 2–10. New York: Pocket Books.

Butler, Jess. 2013. "For White Girls Only? Post Feminism and the Politics of Inclusion." *Feminist Formations* 25 (1): 23–58.

Butler, Judith. 1990. *Gender Trouble: Feminism and the Subversion of Identity*. New York: Routledge.

———. 2004. *Undoing Gender*. New York: Routledge.

Byrd, Ayana and Akiba Solomon 2005. *Naked: Black Women Bare All about their Skin, Hair, Hips, Lips, and Other Parts*. New York: Penguin.

Byrd, Ayana and Lori Tharps. 2014. *Hair Story: Untangling the Roots of Black Hair in America*. New York: Ayana D. Byrd and Lori L. Tharps.

Cairns, Kate, Josée Johnston, and Norah MacKendrick. 2013. "Feeding the 'Organic Child': Mothering through Ethical Consumption." *Journal of Consumer Culture* 13 (2): 97–118.

Calasanti, Toni. 2007. "Bodacious Berry, Potency Wood and the Aging Monster: Gender and Age Relations in Anti-Aging Ads." *Social Forces* 86 (1): 335–355.

Caldwell, Kia. 2007. *Negras in Brazil: Re-envisioning Black Women, Citizenship and the Politics of Identity*. New Brunswick, NJ: Rutgers University Press.

Caldwell, Paulette M. 1991. "Hair Piece: Perspectives on the Intersections of Race and Gender." *Duke Law Journal* 2:365–396.

———. 2008. "Intersectional Bias and the Courts: The Story of *Rogers v. American Airlines*." In *Race Law Stories*, edited by Rachel F. Moran and Devon W. Carbado, 571–600. New York: Foundation Press.

Callahan, Yesha, 2017. "Black Women are Upset over SheaMoisture's New Whitewashing Marketing Ploy." *The Root*. April 27, 2017. Accessed December 21, 2021. www .theroot.com.

Carbado, Devon and Cheryl L. Harris. 2012. "The New Racial Preferences: Rethinking Racial Projects." In *Racial Formation in the 21st Century*, edited by Daniel Martinez HoSang, Oneka LaBennett, and Laura Pulido, 183–212. Berkeley: University of California Press.

Carbado, Devon W. 2013. "Colorblind Intersectionality." *Signs: Journal of Women in Culture and Society* 38 (4): 811–845.

Carney, Nikita. 2016. "All Lives Matter, But So Does Race: Black Lives Matter and the Evolving Role of Social Media." *Humanity and Society* 40 (2): 180–199.

Carr, Leslie. 1997. *"Colorblind" Racism*. Thousand Oaks: SAGE Publications.

Carrington, Ben. 2010. *Race, Sport, and Politics: The Sporting Black Diaspora*. London: SAGE Publications.

Centers for Disease Control and Prevention. 2014. *National Diabetes Statistics Report*. Accessed February 28, 2024 www.cdc.gov.

Cha-Jua, Sundiata Keita. 2001. "Racial Formation and Transformation: Toward a Theory of Black Racial Oppression." *Souls: A Critical Journal of Black Politics, Culture & Society* 3:25–60.

Chang et al. 2022. "Use of Straighteners and other Hair Products and Incident Uterine Cancer." *Journal of the National Cancer Institute* 114 (12): 1636–1645.

Chapkis, Wendy. 1986. *Beauty Secrets*. Boston: South End Press.

Chatelain, Marcia and Kaavya Asoka. 2015. "Women and Black Lives Matter: An Interview with Marcia Chatelain." *Dissent*. www.dissentmagazine.org.

Cherid, Maha Ikram. 2021. "'Ain't Got Enough Money to Pay Me Respect': Blackfishing, Cultural Appropriation, and the Commodification of Blackness." *Critical Studies, Critical Methodologies* 21 (5): 359–364.

Chesebrough, David B. 1998. *Frederick Douglass: Oratory from Slavery*. Westport, CT: Greenwood Press.

Chigumadzi, Panashe. 2016. "White Schools vs. Black Hair in Post-Apartheid South Africa." *New York Times*. October 5, 2016. Accessed December 27, 2021. www.nytimes.com.

Cogan, Jeanine. 1999. "Lesbians Walk the Tightrope of Beauty: Thin Is in but Femme Is Out." *Journal of Lesbian Studies* 3 (4): 77–89.

Collins, Patricia Hill. 1986. "Learning from the Outsider Within: The Sociological Significance of Black Feminist Thought." *Social Problems* 33 (6): S14–S32.

———. 1998. *Fighting Words: Black Women and the Search for Justice*. Minneapolis: University of Minnesota Press.

———. 2000. *Black Feminist Thought: Knowledge, Consciousness, and the Politics of Empowerment*. New York: Routledge.

———. 2005. *Black Sexual Politics: African Americans, Gender, and the New Racism*. New York: Routledge.

Collins, Patricia Hill and Sirma Bilge. 2016. *Intersectionality*. Malden, MA: Polity Press.

Combahee River Collective. (1977) 1995. "A Black Feminist Statement." In *Words of Fire: An Anthology of African American Feminist Thought*, edited by Beverly Guy-Sheftall, 231–240. New York: New Press.

Connell, Raewyn. 2009. *Gender*. Cambridge, UK: Polity Press.

Cooky, Cheryl, Faye Linda Wachs, Michael Messner, and Shari Lee Dworkin. 2010. "It's Not About the Game: Don Imus, Racism and Sexism in Contemporary Media." *Sociology of Sport Journal* 27: 139–159.

Cooper, Brittney. 2017. "SlutWalks vs. Ho Strolls." In *The Crunk Feminist Collection*, edited by Brittney Cooper, Susana Morris, and Robin M. Boylorn, 47–50. New York: Feminist Press.

Craig, Maxine Leeds. 2002. *Ain't I a Beauty Queen?: Black Women, Beauty, and the Politics of Race.* New York: Oxford University Press.

———. 2006. "Race, Beauty, and the Tangled Knot of a Guilty Pleasure." *Feminist Theory* 7 (2): 159–177.

Crais, Clifton and Pamela Scully. 2009. *Sara Baartman and the Hottentot Venus: A Ghost Story and a Biography.* Princeton: Princeton University Press.

Crenshaw, Kimberlé. 1989. "Demarginalizing the Intersection of Race and Sex: A Black Feminist Critique of Antidiscrimination Doctrine, Feminist Theory, and Antiracist Politics." *University of Chicago Legal Forum* 1 (8): 139–167.

———. 1991. "Mapping the Margins: Intersectionality, Identity Politics, and Violence Against Women of Color." *Stanford Law Review* 43 (6): 1241–1299.

Crenshaw, Kimberlé Williams, Andrea J. Ritchie, Rachel Anspach, Rachel Gilmer, and Luke Harris. 2015. "Say Her Name: Resisting Police Brutality Against Black Women." African American Policy Forum & Center for Intersectionality and Social Policy Studies. July 2015. Accessed February 28, 2024. https://www.aapf.org/_files/ugd/62e126_9223ee35c2694ac3bd3f2171504ca3f7.pdf

Cullors, Patrisse. 2018. *When They Call You a Terrorist: A Black Lives Matter Memoir.* New York: St. Martin's Press.

Davis, Angela. 1981. *Women, Race and Class.* New York: Random House.

———. 1994. "Afro Images: Politics, Fashion, and Nostalgia." *Critical Inquiry* 21 (4): 37–45.

Davis, Ebonee. 2016. "Calvin Klein Model Pens Rare and Honest Open Letter to Fashion Industry." *Harper's Bazaar.* July 11, 2016. www.harpersbazaar.com.

———. 2017. "Black Girl Magic in the Fashion Industry." TEDx University of Nevada. www.youtube.com/watch?v=DVJwa06FFIo.

Davis-Sivasothy, Audrey. 2011. *The Science of Black Hair: A Comprehensive Guide to Textured Hair Care.* Stafford, TX: Saja Publishing Company.

———. 2012. *Hair Care Rehab: The Ultimate Hair Repair and Reconditioning Manual.* Stafford, TX: Saja Publishing Company.

———. 2015. *The Science of Transitioning: A Complete Guide to Hair Care for Transitioners and New Naturals.* Stafford, TX: Saja Publishing Company.

De Lucca. Kevin Michael. 1999. "Unruly Arguments: The Body Rhetoric of Earth First!, Act Up, and Queer Nation." *Argumentation and Advocacy* 36 (1): 9–21.

Democratic Alliance. 2016. "Outdated Gauteng School Policies Need to be Reviewed by SGBs." August 29, 2016. Accessed February 28, 2024. https://content.voteda.org/gauteng/2016/08/outdated-gauteng-school-policies-need-to-be-reviewed-by-sgbs/.

Doherty, Philip H. 1987. "Advertising; Essence Bans Ads of Revlon." *New York Times.* January 23, 1987. Accessed February 28, 2024. www.nytimes.com.

Donovan, Maryann, Chandra M Tiwary, Deborah Axelrod, Jannie J. Sasco, Lovell Jones, Richard Hajek, Erin Sauber, Jean Kuo, and Devra, L. Davis. 2007. "Personal Care Products that Contain Estrogens and Xenoestrogens May Increase Breast Cancer Risks." *Medical Hypotheses* 68 (4): 756–766.

Dougan, Laila Lee. 2016. "Policing black women's hair." *Africa Is a Country*. Accessed February 28, 2024. https://africasacountry.com.

Du Bois, W. E. B. 1903. *The Souls of Black Folk*. Chicago: A.C. McClurg & Co.

Duggan, Lisa. 2003. *The Twilight of Equality? Neoliberalism, Cultural Politics, and the Attack on Democracy*. Boston: Beacon Press.

Duke, Bill. 2015. *Light Girls*. Oprah Winfrey Network.

Dworkin, Shari L. and Faye Linda Wachs. 2009. *Body Panic: Gender, Health and the Selling of Fitness*. New York: New York University Press.

Elias, Anna Sofia, Rosalind Gill, and Christina Scharff. 2017. *Aesthetic Labor: Rethinking Beauty Politics in Neoliberalism*. London: Palgrave Macmillan.

Ellington, Tameka. 2014. "Social Networking Sites: A Support System for African American Women Wearing Natural Hair." *International Journal of Fashion Design, Technology and Education* 8 (1): 21–29.

Emerson, Robert, Rachel Fretz, and Linda Shaw. 2011. *Writing Ethnographic Fieldnotes*. Chicago: University of Chicago Press.

Epstein, Samuel S. and Randall Fitzgerald. 2009. *Toxic Beauty: How Cosmetics and Personal Care Products Endanger Your Health, and What You Can Do About It*. Dallas: BenBella Books.

Evans, Adrienne and Sarah Riley. 2013. "Immaculate Consumption: Negotiating the Sex Symbol in Postfeminist Celebrity Culture." *Journal of Gender Studies* 22 (3): 268–281.

Fahs, Breanne. 2011. "Dreaded 'Otherness': Heteronormative Patrolling in Women's Body Hair Rebellions." *Gender & Society* 25 (4): 451–472.

Faludi, Susan. 2009. *Backlash: The Undeclared War Against American Women*. New York: Three Rivers Press.

Falzon, Mark. 2009. *Multi-Sited Ethnography: Theory, Practice, and Locality in Contemporary Research*. Burlington, VT: Ashgate.

Feagin, Joe and Sean Elias. 2013. "Rethinking Racial Formation Theory: A Systemic Racism Critique." *Ethnic and Racial Studies* 36 (6): 931–960.

Federal Bureau of Investigations. August 18, 1970. "Black Panther Party FBI Wanted Poster for Angela Davis." Collection of the Smithsonian National Museum of African American History and Culture. Object 2012.60.8.

Ferguson, Roderick A. 2012. "On the Specificities of Racial Formation: Gender and Sexuality in Historiographies of Race." In *Racial Formation in the Twenty-First Century*, edited by Daniel Martinez HoSang, Oneka LaBennett, and Laura Pulido, 44–56. Berkeley: University of California Press.

Figueiredo, Angela. 1994. "O mercado da boa aparência: as cabeleireiras negras." *Análise & Dados* 3 (4): 33–38.

Finley, Taryn. 2016. "Appeals Court Rules Employers Can Ban Dreadlocks at Work." *Huffington Post*. Accessed February 28, 2024. www.huffpost.com.

Fischer, Ivana. 2020. "A Letter to Black Trans Women About Embracing Our Natural Hair." *Huffington Post*. Accessed February 28, 2024. www.huffpost.com.

Food and Drug Administration. 2022. "Cosmetic Labeling Guide." Accessed February 28, 2024 www.fda.gov.

Ford, Tanisha. 2016. *Liberated Threads: Black Women, Style, and the Global Politics of Soul.* Chapel Hill: University of North Carolina Press.

Foster, Kimberly. (@KimberlyNFoster). 2017. "Black women built SheaMoisture. And not the 'I was teased for having good hair' Black women. Black women will take it right on down too." Twitter, April 24, 2017. https://twitter.com /KimberlyNFoster.

Frank, Jacqueline. 2017. "The Eleventh Circuit Dreadlocks Ban and the Implications of Race Discrimination in the Workplace." *Barry Law Review* 23 (1): 27–40.

Frankel, Mike (@MikeFrankelJSZ). 2018. "Epitome of a team player. A referee wouldn't allow Andrew Johnson of Buena @brhschiefs to wrestle with a cover over his dreadlocks. It was either an impromptu haircut, or a forfeit. Johnson chose the haircut, then won by sudden victory in OT to help spark Buena to a win." Twitter, December 20, 2018, 11:54 a.m. https://twitter.com/MikeFrankelSNJ/status /1075811774954463235.

Fuller, Gillian. 2015. "Teen Vogue Slammed for Using Light Skinned Models in African Braids Article." Elite Daily. June 23, 2015. www.elitedaily.com.

Gaard, Greta. 2010. "Ecofeminism and Native American Cultures: Pushing the Limits of Cultural Imperialism?" In *Ecofeminism: Women, Animals, Nature*, edited by Greta Gaard, 295–314. Philadelphia: Temple University Press.

Gaines, Kevin. 1996. *Uplifting the Race: Black Leadership, Politics, and Culture in the Twentieth Century.* Chapel Hill: University of North Carolina Press.

Garland-Thomson, Rosemarie. 1996. *Freakery: Cultural Spectacles of the Extraordinary Body.* New York: Columbia University Press.

Gibson-Wood, Hilary and Sarah Wakefield. 2013. "'Participation,' White Privilege and Environmental Justice: Understanding Environmentalism Among Hispanics in Toronto." *Antipode* 45 (3): 641–62.

Gilkes, Cheryl Townsend. 1983. "From Slavery to Social Welfare: Racism and the Control of Black Women." In *Class, Race, and Sex: The Dynamics of Control*, edited by Amy Swerdlow and Johanna Lessinger, 288–300. Boston: G. K. Hall.

Gill, Rosalind. 2007. *Gender and the Media.* Malden, NY: Polity Press.

———. 2021. "Neoliberal Beauty." In *The Routledge Companion to Beauty Politics*, edited by Maxine Leeds Craig, 9–18. New York: Routledge.

Gill, Rosalind and Christina Sharff. 2011. *New Femininities: Postfeminism, Neoliberalism and Subjectivity.* Basingstoke, UK: Palgrave Macmillan.

Gill, Tiffany M. 2001. "'I Had My Own Business . . . So I Didn't Have to Worry': Beauty Salons, Beauty Culturists, and the Politics of African American Female Entrepreneurship." In *Beauty and Business: Commerce, Gender, and Culture in Modern America*, edited by Philip Scranton, 92–111. New York: Routledge.

———. 2010. *Beauty Shop Politics: African American Women's Activism in the Beauty Industry.* Chicago: University of Illinois Press.

———. 2015. "#TeamNatural: Black Hair and the Politics of Community in Digital Media." *Journal of Contemporary African Art* 37:70–79.

Gilroy, Paul. 1993. *The Black Atlantic: Modernity and Double Consciousness*. London: Verso.

Glenn, Evelyn Nakano. 1999. "The Social Construction and Institutionalization of Race and Gender: An Integrative Framework." In *Revisioning Gender*, edited by Myra Marx Feree, Judith Lorber, and Beth B. Hess, 3–43. Walnut Creek, CA: AltaMira Press.

———. 2008. "Yearning for Lightness: Transnational Circuits in the Marketing and Consumption of Skin Lighteners." *Gender and Society* 22 (3): 281–302.

Green, Toby. 2012. *The Rise of the Trans-Atlantic Slave Trade in Western Africa, 1300–1589*. New York: Cambridge University Press.

Guy, Taren. (@Auset_ntru). August 30, 2016. "Dear Natural Hair Community." [Instagram Post, August 30, 2016.]. Retrieved https://www.instagram.com/p/BJwBoabAQjB/?hl=en.

Guy-Sheftall, Beverly, ed. 1995. *Words of Fire: An Anthology of African American Feminist Thought*. New York: The New Press.

Haiken, Elizabeth. 2000. "The Making of the Modern Face: Cosmetic Surgery." *Social Research* 67 (1): 81–97.

Hallett, Ronald and Kristen Barber. 2014. "Ethnographic Research in a Cyber Era." *Journal of Contemporary Ethnography* 43 (3): 306–330.

Hancock, Ange Marie. 2004. *The Politics of Disgust: The Public Identity of the Welfare Queen*. New York: New York University Press.

Harris, Cheryl L. 1993. "Whiteness as Property." *Harvard Law Review* 106 (8): 1707–1791.

Haug, Frigga. 1987. *Female Sexualization: Questions for Feminism*. London: Verso.

Hays, Sharon. 2004. *Flat Broke with Children: Women in the Age of Welfare Reform*. New York: Oxford University Press.

Heller, Chaia. 2010. "For the Love of Nature: Ecology and the Cult of the Romantic." In *Ecofeminism: Women, Animals, Nature*, edited by Greta Gaard, 219–242. Philadelphia: Temple University Press.

Herzig, Rebecca M. 2016. *Plucked: A History of Hair Removal*. New York: New York University Press.

Higginbotham, Evelyn. 1993. *Righteous Discontent: The Women's Movement in the Black Baptist Church, 1880–1920*. Cambridge: Harvard University Press.

Hochschild, Jennifer L. and Vesla Weaver. 2007. "The Skin Color Paradox and the American Racial Order." *Social Forces* 86 (2): 643–670.

Hofman, Katen and Aviva Tugendhaft. 2016. "South Africans have a Sweet Tooth So Shouldn't Say No to a Sugar Tax." *The Conversation*. August 25, 2016. Accessed December 14, 2016. https://theconversation.com.

hooks, bell. 1984. *Feminist Theory: From Margin to Center*. Boston: South End Press.

———. 2014. *Ain't I a Woman: Black Women and Feminism*. New York: Routledge.

————. 2015a. *Black Looks: Race and Representation*. New York: Routledge.

————. 2015b. *Sisters of the Yam: Black Women and Self-Recovery*. New York: Routledge.

hooks, bell and Cornel West. 1991. *Breaking Bread: Insurgent Black Intellectual Life*. Boston: South End Press.

Hordge-Freeman, Elizabeth. 2015. *The Color of Love: Racial Features Stigma, and Socialization in Black Brazilian Families*. Austin: University of Texas Press.

Howze, Candace. 2017. "Free Yo Edges." *CRWN Magazine* 1(2): 120–121.

Hull, Gloria T., Batricia Bell-Scott, and Barbara Smith. 1982. *All the Women are White, All the Blacks are Men, But Some of Us are Brave*. New York: Feminist Press.

Hunter, Margaret. 2005. *Race, Gender, and the Politics of Skin Tone*. New York: Routledge.

Jacobs-Huey, Lanita. 2006. *From the Kitchen to the Parlor: Language and Becoming in African American Women's Hair Care*. New York: Oxford University Press.

James-Todd, Tamarra, Mary Beth Terry, Janet Rich-Edwards, Andrea Deierlein, and Riny Senie. 2011. "Childhood Hair Product Use and Earlier Age at Menarche in a Racially Diverse Study Population: A Pilot Study." *Annals of Epidemiology* 21 (6): 461–465.

Jarrin, Alvaro. 2016. "Towards a Biopolitics of Beauty: Eugenics, Aesthetic Hierarchies and Plastic Surgery in Brazil." *Journal of Latin American Cultural Studies* 24 (4): 535–552.

Jha, Meeta. 2015. *The Global Beauty Industry: Colorism, Racism and the National Body*. Florence: Taylor and Francis.

Jerkins, Morgan. 2017. "The White Washing of Natural Hair Care Lines." *Racked*. April 5, 2017. Accessed December 27, 2021. www.racked.com.

Johnson, Chelsea. 2015. "'Just Because I Dance Like a Ho I'm Not a Ho': Cheerleading at the Intersection of Race, Class and Gender." *Sociology of Sport Journal* 32 (4): 377–394.

————. 2016. "Black Beauty and the Economics of Liberation." *CRWN Magazine*, 1(1): 48–50.

————. 2016. "Kinky, Curly Hair: A Tool of Resistance Across the African Diaspora." *The Conversation*. Retrieved from https://theconversation.com.

————. 2016. "My Natural, My Politics, My Way." *CRWN Magazine*, 1(1): 4–7.

————. 2017. "Bossiekop is Beautiful," *CRWN Magazine*, 1(2):133–134.

————. 2017. "How 'Beauty Myths' are Holding Women Back Today." *Naturally Curly*. www.naturallycurly.com.

————. 2017. "What It's Like Having Natural Hair in South Africa #CurlsAroundTheWorld." *Naturally Curly*. www.naturallycurly.com.

————. 2018. "10 Books by Academics That Will Change the Way You Think About Hair." *Naturally Curly*. www.naturallycurly.com.

————. 2018. "The History of Headwraps: Then, There and Now." *Naturally Curly*. www.naturallycurly.com.

———. 2018. "What Your Hair Really Says About You, According to Scholars of the Body." *Naturally Curly*. www.naturallycurly.com.

Johnson, Chelsea and Kristen Barber. 2019. "The Gender and Sexual Politics of Hair: The Modern Age: 1920–2000+" in *A Cultural History of Hair*, edited by Geraldine Biddle-Perry, pp. 111-128. New York: Bloomsbury.

Johnson, Elizabeth. 2013. *Resistance and Empowerment in Black Women's Hair Styling*. Burlington, VT: Ashgate Publishing Company.

Johnson, E. Patrick. 2003. *Appropriating Blackness: Performance and the Politics of Authenticity*. Durham, NC: Duke University Press.

Jones, I. S. 2016. "Wild Crown." *Matador Review: A Quarterly Missive of Alternative Concern*. Summer 2016.

Kandaswamy, Priya. 2012. "Gendering Racial Formation." In *Racial Formation in the Twenty-First Century*, edited by Daniel Martinez HoSang, Oneka LaBennett, and Laura Pulido, 23–43. Berkeley: University of California Press.

Kang, Miliann. 2003. "The Managed Hand: The Commercialization of Bodies and Emotions in Korean-Immigrant Owned Nail Salons." *Gender and Society* 17 (6): 820–839.

———. 2010. *The Managed Hand: Race, Gender, and the Body in Beauty Service Work*. Berkeley: University of California Press.

Kauer, Karrie. 2016. "Yoga Culture and Neoliberal Embodiment of Health." In *Yoga, The Body, and Embodied Social Change: An Intersectional Feminist Analysis* edited by Beth Berila, Melanie Klein, and Chelsea Jackson Roberts, 91–108. Lanham, MD: Lexington Books.

Kaw, Eugenia. 1993. "Medicalization of Racial Features: Asian American Women and Cosmetic Surgery." *Medical Anthropology Quarterly* 7 (1): 74–89.

Kelley, Robin. 1997. "Nap Time: Historicizing the Afro." *Fashion Theory* 1 (4): 339–351.

Kim, Claire Jean. 1999. "The Racial Triangulation of Asian Americans." *Politics Society* 27 (1): 105–138.

King, Shaun. (@shaunking). 2018. "Disgusting and heartbreaking. A referee known for his racism, Alan Maloney (google him), made high school wrestler Andrew Johnson cut off his dreads or lose the match. They were covered and gave him no advantage. So he cut them off. He won the match. But this never should've been allowed." Instagram photo, December 21, 2018, Account permanently deleted.

King-O'Riain, Rebecca Chiyoko. 2006. *Pure Beauty: Judging Race in Japanese American Beauty Pageants*. Minneapolis: University of Minnesota Press.

Kitch, Sally. 2009. *The Specter of Sex: Gendered Foundations of Racial Formation in the United States*. Albany: State University of New York Press.

Knowles, Solange and Sampha Sisay. 2016. "Don't Touch My Hair." *A Seat at the Table*. Columbia Records.

Ko, Alph. 2014. "Can White Women be a Part of the Natural Hair Space?" *Natural Hair Mag*. July 3, 2014. Accessed July 4, 2015. www.naturalhairmag.com.

Koval, Christy Zhou and Ashley Shelby Rosette. 2021. "The Natural Hair Bias in Job Recruitment." *Social Psychological & Personality Science* 12 (5): 741–750.

Krudy, Edward. 2016. "Justice Department Opens Criminal Probe into Black Louisiana Man's Death." Reuters. July 6, 2016. www.reuters.com.

Lake, Obiagele. 2003. *Blue Veins and Kinky Hair: Naming and Color Consciousness in African America*. Westport, CT: Praeger.

Laslett, Barbara and Barrie Thorne. 1997. *Feminist Sociology: Life Histories of a Movement*. New Brunswick, NJ: Rutgers University Press.

Lau, Kimberly J. 2011. "New Bodies of Knowledge" In *Body Language: Sisters in Shape, Black Women's Fitness and Feminist Identity Politics*, edited by Kimberly J. Lau, 107–142. Philadelphia: Temple University Press.

Lebron, Christopher J. 2017. *The Making of Black Lives Matter: A Brief History of an Idea*. New York: Oxford University Press.

Lee, Spike, dir. 1988. *School Daze*. 40 Acres and A Mule Filmworks.

Leem, So Yeon. 2016. "The Dubious Enhancement: Making South Korea a Plastic Surgery Nation." *East Asian Science, Technology and Society* 10 (1): 51–71.

Lemire, Beverly. 2018. *Global Trade and the Transformation of Consumer Cultures*. Cambridge: Cambridge University Press.

Lesnik-Oberstein, Karin. 2013. *The Last Taboo: Women and Body Hair*. Manchester, UK: Manchester University Press.

Lewis, Jioni, Marlene Williams, Erica Peppers and Cecile Gadson. 2017. "Applying Intersectionality to Explore the Relations Between Gendered Racism and Health Among Black Women." *Journal of Counseling Psychology* 64 (5): 475–486.

Light, Ivan H. and Edna Bonacich. 1988. *Immigrant Entrepreneurs: Koreans in Los Angeles, 1965–1982*. Berkeley: University of California Press.

Lipsitz, George. 1994. "We Know What Time It Is: Race, Class and Youth Culture in the Nineties." In *Microfone Fiends: Youth Music and Youth Culture*, edited by A. Ross and Tricia Rose, 17–28. New York: Routledge.

———. 2006. *The Possessive Investment in Whiteness: How White People Profit from Identity Politics*. Philadelphia: Temple University Press.

L'Oréal. 2014. "L'Oréal USA Signs Agreement to Acquire Carol's Daughter." October 20, 2014. Accessed ____. www.lorealusa.com.

Lorde, Audre. 1984. *Sister Outsider*. Berkeley: Crossing Press.

———. 1988. *A Burst of Light: Essays*. Ithaca, NY: Firebrand Books.

Lowe, Lisa. 1996. *Immigrant Acts: On Asian American Cultural Politics*. Durham, NC: Duke University Press.

Luders-Manuel. 2015. "The Mixed-Race Community's Response to Rachel Dolezal." Skirt Collective. June 16, 2015. Accessed June 20, 2015. http://t.co/DskN2OpXVX?amp=1.

Lyle, Jennifer, Jeanell Jones, and Gail Drakes. 1999. "Beauty on the Borderland: On Being Black Lesbian and Beautiful." *Journal of Lesbian Studies* 3 (4): 45–53.

Ma, Chun-Lung. 2021. "Negotiating Chineseness through English Dialects in *Crazy Rich Asians*." In *Contesting Chineseness: Ethnicity, Identity, and Nation in China and Southeast Asia*, edited by Chang-Yau Hoon and Ying-kit Chan, 223–237. Germany: Springer Singapore.

MacKendrick, Norah. 2014. "More Work for Mother: Chemical Body Burdens as a Maternal Responsibility." *Gender & Society* 28 (5): 705–728.

Mahr, Krista. 2016. "White Schools vs. Black Hair in Post-Apartheid South Africa." *Washington Post*. September 3, 2016. www.washingtonpost.com.

Makalintal, Bettina. 2020. "Awkwafina's Past Hakes Her a Complicated Icon of Asian American Representation." *Vice*. January 24, 2020. Accessed December 27, 2021. www.vice.com.

Mann, Susan. 2011. "Pioneers of U.S. Ecofeminism and Environmental Justice." *Feminist Formations* 23 (2): 1–25.

Marques, Leonardo. 2016. *The United States and the Transatlantic Slave Trade to the Americas, 1776–1867*. New Haven: Yale University Press.

McAndrew, Malia. 2010. "A Twentieth Century Triangle Trade: Selling Black Beauty at Home and Abroad, 1945–1965." *Enterprise & Society* 11 (4): 784–807.

McCall, Leslie. 2005. "The Complexity of Intersectionality," *Signs: Journal of Women in Culture and Society* 30:1771–1800.

McCarthy, John and Mayer Zald. 1977. "Resource Mobilization and Social Movements: A Partial Theory." *American Journal of Sociology* 82:1212–1241.

McCaughey, Martha. 1998. "The Fighting Spirit: Women's Self-Defense Training and the Discourse of Sexed Embodiment." *Gender & Society* 12 (3): 277–300.

McGill Johnson, Alexis, Rachel D. Godsil, Jessical MacFarlane, Linda Tropp, and Phillip Atiba Goff. 2017. "The 'Good Hair' Study: Explicit and Implicit Attitudes Towards Black Women's Hair." The Perception Institute. Accessed Jan. 1, 2021. https://perception.org.

McIntosh, Peggy. 1989. "White Privilege: Unpacking the Invisible Knapsack." *Peace and Freedom Magazine*, July/August, 1989: 10-12.

McLaughlin, Kelly and Mia De Graaf. 2017. "So THAT'S How She Does It! Rachel Dolezal 'Gets Regular Spray Tans for $60 a Month' and Wears a Weave to Maintain her Black Identity." *Daily Mail*. June 15, 2017. Accessed December 27, 2021. www .dailymail.co.uk.

McRobbie, Angela. 2009. *The Aftermath of Feminism: Gender, Culture and Social Change*. London: Sage Publications.

Mears, Ashley. 2011. *Pricing Beauty: The Making of a Fashion Model*. Berkeley: University of California Press.

Melosi, Martin. 2006. "Environmental Justice, Ecoracism, and Environmental History." In *To Know the Wind and the Rain: African Americans and Environmental History*, edited by Dianne D. Glave and Mark Stoll, 120–132. Pittsburgh: University of Pittsburgh Press.

Mercer, Kobena. 1994. *Welcome to the Jungle: New Positions in Black Cultural Studies.* Cambridge, MA: The MIT Press.

Merianos, Ashley, Rebecca Vidourek, and Keith King. 2013. "Medicalization of Female Beauty: A Content Analysis of Cosmetic Procedures." *The Qualitative Report* 18 (4): 1–14.

Meyer, David S. and Nancy Whittier. 1994. "Social Movement Spillover." *Social Problems* 41 (2): 277.

Miles, Tiya. 2018. "Black Hair's Blockbuster Moment." *New York Times*, February 23, 2018. www.nytimes.com.

Mitchell, Michelle. 2004. *Righteous Propagation: African Americans and the Politics of Racial Destiny after Reconstruction.* Chapel Hill: University of North Carolina Press.

Moore, Mignon. 2006. "Lipstick or Timberlands? Meanings of Gender Presentation in Black Lesbian Communities." *Signs: Journal of Women in Culture and Society* 32 (1): 113–139.

Moraga, Cherríe and Gloria Anzaldúa. 1983. *This Bridge Called My Back: Writings by Radical Women of Color.* New York: Kitchen Table, Women of Color Press.

Morrison, Angeline. 2006. "Black Skin, Big Hair; Cultural Appropriation of the 'Afro.'" In *Image into Identity: Constructing and Assigning Identity in a Culture of Modernity*, edited by Michael Wintle, 101–118. Amsterdam: Rodopi.

Morrison, Toni. 1970. *The Bluest Eye.* New York: Holt, Rinehart and Winston, Inc.

Morrow, Willie Lee. 1973. *400 Years Without a Comb.* San Diego: Black Publishers of San Diego.

Nagel, Joane. 2003. *Race, Ethnicity, and Sexuality: Intimate Intersections, Forbidden Frontiers.* New York: Oxford University Press.

Ng, Serena and Ryan Dezember. 2015. "Bain Capital to Take Minority Stake in Sundial Brands." *Wall Street Journal.* September 2, 2015. www.wsj.com.

Nicholson, Greg. 2016. "South African Student Speak Out Against 'Aggressive' Ban on Afro Hair." *Guardian.* August 31, 2016. Accessed December 27, 2021. www.theguardian.com.

Nielsen Company. 2017. "African American Women: Our Science, Her Magic." Accessed December 27, 2021. www.nielsen.com.

O'Connor, Anahad. 2011. "Surgeon General Calls for Health Over Hair." *New York Times.* August 25, 2011. Accessed December 26, 2021. well.blogs.nytimes.com.

Oluo, Ijeoma. 2017. "The Heart of Whiteness: Ijeoma Oluo Interviews Rachel Dolezal, the Woman Who Identifies as Black." The Stranger. April 19, 2017. Accessed February 28, 2024. www.thestranger.com.

Omi, Michael and Howard Winant. 1994. *Racial Formation in the United States: From the 1960s to the 1990s.* New York: Routledge.

———. 2012. "Conclusion: Racial Formation Rules: Continuity, Instability and Change." In *Racial Formation in the Twenty-First Century*, edited by Daniel Martinez HoSang, Oneka LaBennett, and Laura Pulido, 302–332. Berkeley: University of California Press.

Opiah, Antonia. 2013. "You Can Touch My Hair: What Were We Thinking?!" *Huffington Post*. June 18, 2013. www.huffpost.com.

———. 2013. "You Can Touch My Hair." Un-Ruly.com. October 20, 2013. Accessed February 28, 2023. https://www.un-ruly.com.

Parker, Bashiera. 2020. "Short Back and Sides, No Afros Please . . ." News24. Accessed December 27, 2021. www.news24.com.

Patrice, Christina. 2014. "Beauty Conglomerate L'Oreal, a Company with a Troubled History with Black Women, Buys Out Carol's Daughter." *Black Girl with Long Hair*. October 21, 2014. https://bglh-marketplace.com.

Pergament, Danielle. 2015. "You (Yes, You) Can Have an Afro.*" *Allure*. August 2015.

Peterson, Abby. 2001. "The Militant Body and Political Communication: The Medialisation of Violence." In *Contemporary Political Protest: Essays on Political Militancy*, edited by ____, 69–101. Aldershot, UK: Ashgate.

Pichardo, Nelson. 1997. "New Social Movements: A Critical Review." *Annual Review of Sociology* 23 (1): 411–430.

Pierce, Chester. 1970. "Offensive Mechanisms." In *The Black Seventies*, edited by F. B. Barbour, 265–282 .Boston, MA: Porter Sargent.

Pixel, Momo. 2017. *Hair Nah*. Accessed December 27, 2017. www.hairnah.com.

Plumwood, Val. 1993. *Feminism and the Mastery of Nature*. London: Routledge.

Polletta, Francesca and James M. Jasper. 2001. "Collective Identity and Social Movements." *Annual Review of Sociology* 27:283–305.

Portes, Alejandro and Leif Jensen. 1989. "The Enclave and the Entrants: Patterns of Ethnic Enterprise in Miami before and after Mariel." *American Sociological Review* 54 (6): 929–949.

Posel, Deborah. 2001a. "Race as Common Sense: Racial Classification in 20th Century South Africa." *African Studies Review* 44 (2): 87–114.

———. 2001b. "What's in a Name? Racial Categorisations Under Apartheid and their Afterlife." *Transformation: Critical Perspectives on Southern Africa* 47:50–74.

"'Racist School Hair Rules' Suspended at SA's Pretoria Girl's High." 2016. BBC News, August 30, 2016. Accessed December 27, 2021, www.bbc.com.

Ransby, Barbara. 2018. *Making All Black Lives Matter: Reimagining Freedom in the Twenty-First Century*. Berkeley: University of California Press.

Rawley, James A. and Stephen D. Behrendt. 2005. *The Transatlantic Slave Trade: A History*. Lincoln: University of Nebraska Press.

Reese, Hope. 2018. "Chimamanda Ngozi Adichie: I Became Black in America." JSTOR Daily. August 29, 2018. Accessed December 28, 2021. https://daily.jstor.org.

Riley, Shamara Shantu. 2004. "Ecology is a Sistah's Issue Too: The Politics of Emergent Afrocentric Ecowomanism." In *This Sacred Earth: Religion, Nature, Environment*, edited by Roger S. Gottelib, 428–437. New York: Routledge.

Roberts, Dorothy. (1997) 2016. *Killing the Black Body: Race, Reproduction and the Meaning of Liberty*. New York: Vintage.

Roberts, Tanya. 2014. "5 Trends Set to Shape the Black Haircare Market in the Next 5 Years." Mintel. Accessed February 28, 2024. www.mintel.com.

Robinson, Phoebe. 2016. *You Can't Touch My Hair and Other Things I Still have to Explain.* New York: Plume.

Rooks, Noliwe M. 1996. *Hair Raising: Beauty, Culture, and African American Women.* New Brunswick, NJ: Rutgers University Press.

Rose, Tricia. 1994. *Black Noise: Rap Music and Black Culture in Contemporary America.* Middletown, CT: Wesleyan University Press.

Rosenberg L., Boggs D. A., Adams-Campbell L. L., and Palmer J. R. 2007. "Hair Relaxers Not Associated with Breast Cancer Risk: Evidence from the Black Women's Health Study." *Cancer Epidemiology, Biomarkers & Prevention* 16 (5): 1035–1037.

Roth, Benita. 2004. *Separate Roads to Feminism: Black, Chicana, and White Feminist Movements in America's Second Wave.* Cambridge: Cambridge University Press.

Rowe, Kristin Denise. 2021. "Beyond 'Becky with the Good Hair': Hair, Beauty, and Interiority in Beyoncé Knowles Carters' 'Sorry.'" In *Beyoncé in the World: Making Meaning with Queen Bey in Troubled Times*, edited by Christina Baade and Kristin McGee, 341–367. Middletown, CT: Wesleyan University Press.

———. 2021. "Rooted: On Black Women, Beauty, Hair, and Embodiment." In *The Routledge Companion to Beauty Politics*, edited by Maxine Leeds Craig, 186–204. New York: Routledge.

Rupp, Leila J. and Verta Taylor. 1999. "Forging Feminist Identity in an International Movement: A Collective Identity Approach to Twentieth-Century Feminism." *Signs: Journal of Women in Culture and Society* 24 (2): 363–386.

Russell-Cole, Kathy, Midge Wilson, and Ronald E. Hall. 1993. *The Color Complex: The Politics of Skin Color Among African Americans.* New York: Anchor Books.

———. 2013. *The Color Complex: The Politics of Skin Color in a New Millennium.* New York: Anchor Books.

Saint Heron. October 7, 2016. "A Seat with Us: A Conversation Between Solange Knowles, Mrs. Tina Lawson, & Judnick Mayard." https://saintheron.com.

Salhotra, Pooja. 2024. "Judge says Texas school district can punish Black student for length of his hairstyle." Texas Tribune. February 22, 2024. https://texastribune.org.

Samanga, Rufaro. 2017. "Why Racist Policies in South African Schools Go Beyond Just Hair." *OkayAfrica.* Accessed December 27, 2021. www.okayafrica.com.

Sanchez, Sonia. 1970. "blk/rhetoric." In *We a BaddDDD People*, 15–16. Detroit: Broadside Press.

Sander, Courtnay. 2000. "Dyeing for Grey Hair." *Global Cosmetic Industry* 166:28–33.

Saro-Wiwa, Zina. 2012. "Black Women's Transitions to Natural Hair." *New York Times.* May 21, 2012. www.nytimes.com.

Sasson-Levy, Orna and Tamar Rapoport. 2003. "Body, Gender, and Knowledge in Protest Movements: The Israeli Case." *Gender & Society* 17 (3): 379–403.

Sebambo, Khumo. 2016. "Azania House as a Symbol of the Black Imagination." *The Salon: The Johannesburg Workshop in Theory and Criticism* 9:108–110.

Settler, Henrietta Monica. 2017. "'Hair Economies': Power and Ethics in an Ethno-graphic Study of Female African Hairdressers in Cape Town." Master's thesis, Department of Social Science Methods, Stellenbosch University.

SheaMoisture (@sheamoisture). 2017. "Wow—we really f-ed this one up! Please know that our intent was not, & would never be, to disrespect our commu-nity." Twitter, April 24, 2015, 4:07 p.m. https://twitter.com/SheaMoisture/status /856615548767145985.

Shumway, Rebecca. 2011. *The Fante and the Transatlantic Slave Trade.* Rochester, NY: University of Rochester Press.

Silverman, Robert M. 2000. *Doing Business in Minority Markets: Black and Korean En-trepreneurs in Chicago's Ethnic Beauty Aids Industry.* New York: Garland Publishing.

Smith, Zadie. 2000. *White Teeth.* New York: Vintage International.

Springer, Kimberly. 2007. "Divas, Evil Black Bitches, and Bitter Black Women: African American women in Postfeminist and Post-Civil Rights Popular Culture." In *Inter-rogating Postfeminism*, edited by D. Negra and Y. Tasker, 249–276. Durham, NC: Duke University Press.

Stein, Arlene. 1997. *Sex and Sensibility: Stories of a Lesbian Generation.* Berkeley: Uni-versity of California Press.

Stenberg, Amandla. 2015. "Don't Cash Crop My Cornrows." YouTube, uploaded by Hype Hair Magazine (@hypehairmag). April 15, 2015. www.youtube.com/watch?v =O1KJRRSB_XA.

Stevens, Wesley. 2021. "Blackfishing on Instagram: Influencing and the Commodifica-tion of Black Urban Aesthetics." *Social Media & Society* 7 (3).

Stiel, Laura, Paris B. Adkins-Jackson, Phyllis Clark, Eudora Mitchell, and Susane Mont-gomery. 2016. "A Review of Hair Product Use on Breast Cancer Risk in African American Women." *Cancer Medicine* 5 (3): 597–604.

Stille, Darlene R. 2007. *Madam C. J. Walker: Entrepreneur and Millionaire.* Minneapo-lis, MN: Compass Point Books.

Stilson, Jeff, dir. 2009. *Chris Rock's Good Hair.* Chris Rock Entertainment and HBO Films. DVD.

Sturgeon, Noël. 1997. *Ecofeminist Natures: Race, Gender, Feminist Theory and Political Action.* New York: Routledge.

Sue, Derald Wing. 2010. *Microaggressions in Everyday Life: Race, Gender, and Sexual Orientation.* Hoboken, NJ: John Wiley & Sons.

Sudbury, Julia. 2010. "(Re)constructing Multiracial Blackness: Women's Activism, Dif-ference and Collective Identity in Britain." *Ethnic and Racial Studies* 24 (1): 29–49.

Sunderland, Mitchell. 2015. "In Rachel Dolezal's Skin." Vice. February 28, 2024. https://www.vice.com/en/article/gvz79j/rachel-dolezal-profile-interview.

Sundial Brands. 2015. "10 Reasons We Chose a New Partner." September 2, 2015. Ac-cessed September 3, 2015. www.sundialbrands.com.

Sutton, Barbara. 2010. *Bodies in Crisis: Culture, Violence, and Women's Resistance in Neoliberal Argentina.* New Brunswick, NJ: Rutgers University Press.

Synnott, Anthony. 1993. *The Body Social: Symbolism, Self and Society*. London: Routledge.

Tate, Shirley. 2007. "Black Beauty: Shade, Hair and Anti-Racist Aesthetics." *Ethnic and Racial Studies* 30 (2): 300–319.

———. 2017. *The Governmentality of Black Beauty Shame: Discourse, Iconicity and Resistance*. London: Palgrave.

———. 2021. "'I Do Not See Myself as Anything Else than White': Black Resistance to Racial Cosplay Blackfishing." In *The Routledge Companion to Beauty Politics*, edited by Maxine Leeds Craig, 205–226. New York: Routledge.

Tate, Candis F. 2016. "Loving Blackness: Black Women Digital Content Creators and the Transformative Healing Powers of the Contemporary Natural Hair Movement." Master's thesis, Department of Communications, Wake Forest University.

Taylor, Dorceta E. 1997. "Women of Color, Environmental Justice, and Ecofeminism." In *Ecofeminism: Women, Culture, Nature*, edited by Karen Warren and Nisvan Erkal, 38–81. Bloomington: University of Indiana Press.

Taylor, Keeanga-Yamahtta. 2016. *From #BlackLivesMatter to Black Liberation*. Chicago: Haymarket Books.

Taylor, Verta and Nancy Whittier. 1999. "Collective Identity in Social Movement Communities: Lesbian Feminist Mobilization." In *Waves of Protest: Social Movements Since the Sixties*, edited by Jo Freeman and Victoria Johnson, 169–195. Lanham, MD: Rowman & Littlefield.

Thompson, Cheryl. 2009. "Black Women, Beauty, and Hair as a Matter of *Being*." *Women's Studies* 38:831–856.

Tinsley, Omise'eke. 2018. *Beyoncé in Formation: Remixing Black Feminism*. Austin: University of Texas Press.

Tiwary, Chandra M. 1998. "Premature Sexual Development in Children Following the Use of Estrogen- or Placenta-Containing Hair Products." *Clinical Pediatrics* 37 (12): 733–739.

Truth, Sojourner. (1867) 2011. "When Woman Gets Her Rights Man Will Be Right." In *Words of Fire: An Anthology of African-American Feminist Thought*, edited by Beverly Guy-Sheftall, 37–38. New York: The New Press.

Ture, Kwame and Charles V. Hamilton. (1967) 1992. *Black Power: The Politics of Liberation in America*. New York: Vintage Books.

Twine, France Winddance. 1998. *Racism in a Racial Democracy: The Maintenance of White Supremacy in Brazil*. New Brunswick, NJ: Rutgers University Press.

US Democratic Town Hall in Columbia, South Carolina. Aired February 23, 2016 on CNN.

US Department of Health and Human Services Office of Minority Health. 2017. "Profile: Black/African Americans." Accessed April 25, 2017. https://minorityhealth.hhs.gov.

US General Accounting Office. 2000. "Better Targeting of Airline Passengers Could Produce Better Results." US Customs Service. Accessed Jan. 1, 2021. www.gao.gov.

Victor, Ojakorotu and Esuola Olukayode Segun. 2016. "FeesMustFall: The 'Inner' Gender Dimensions and Implications for Political Participation in South Africa." *Gender & Behaviour* 14 (2): 7185–7190.

Walker, Alice. 1983. *In Search of Our Mothers' Gardens*. Orlando, FL: Harvest Books.

———. 1989. "Oppressed Hair Puts a Ceiling on the Brain." In *Living by the Work: Essays,* 69–74. San Diego: Harvard Brace Jovanovich.

Walker, Juliet E. 2009. *The History of Black Business in America: Capitalism, Race and Entrepreneurship*. Chapel Hill: University of North Carolina Press.

Walker, Susannah. 2000. "Black Is Profitable: The Commodification of the Afro, 1960–1975." *Enterprise & Society* 1 (3): 536–564.

———. 2007. *Style and Status: Selling Beauty to African American Women, 1920–1975*. Lexington: University Press of Kentucky.

Wallace, Michelle. 1990. *Black Macho and the Myth of the Superwoman*. New York: Verso.

Warren, Dorian. 2015. "Rachel Dolezal and Race as a Social Construct." Nerding Out, MSNBC. June 17, 2015. www.msnbc.com.

Weitz, Rose. 2005. *Rapunzel's Daughters: What Women's Hair Tells Us about Women's Lives*. New York: Farrar, Straus and Giroux.

———. 2009. "A History of Women's Bodies." In *The Politics of Women's Bodies: Sexuality, Appearance, and Behavior,* Third Edition, 3–12. New York: Oxford University Press.

West, Candace and Don H. Zimmerman. 1987. "Doing Gender." *Gender & Society* 1 (2): 125–151.

West, Candace and Sarah Fenstermaker 1995. "Doing Difference." *Gender & Society* 9 (1): 8–37.

White, Brooklyn. 2024. "Beyoncé, the Boss." Essence. February 23, 2024. www.essence.com.

Willett, Julie. 2000. *Permanent Waves: The Making of the American Beauty Shop*. New York: New York University Press.

Winfrey, Oprah, Tracee Ellis Ross, Michaela Angela Davis, Raeshem Nijhon, Carri Twigg and Kisha Imani Cameron. 2022. *The Hair Tales*. Culture House, Joy Mill Entertainment, Tetravision and Harpo Films.

Wingfield, Adia Harvey. 2008. *Doing Business with Beauty: Black Women, Hair Salons, and the Racial Enclave Economy*. Lanham, MD: Rowman & Littlefield.

Wise, Lauren, Julie R. Palmer, David Reich, Yvette C. Cozier, and Lynn Rosenberg. 2012. "Hair Relaxer Use and Risk of Uterine Leiomyomata in African American Women." *American Journal of Epidemiology* 175 (5): 432–440.

Witz, Anne. 2000. "Whose Body Matters? Feminist Sociology and the Corporeal Turn in Sociology and Feminism." *Body & Society* 6(1): 1–24.

Wolf, Naomi. 1991. *The Beauty Myth: How Images of Beauty are Used Against Women*. New York: Morrow.

Woolford, Susan J., Carole Woolford-Hunt, Sami Areej, Natalie Blake, and David Williams. 2016. "No Sweat: African American Adolescent Girls' Opinions of Hairstyle Choices and Physical Activity." *BMC Obesity* 3 (1): 31–38.

Work Projects Administration. 1936. *Federal Writers' Project: Slave Narrative Project*, vol. 16, Texas, Part 3, Lewis-Ryles. Library of Congress. www.loc.gov.

X, Malcolm and Alex Haley. 1964. *The Autobiography of Malcolm X*. New York: Random House.

Yancey, George. 2016. *Black Bodies, White Gazes: The Continuing Significance of Race in America*. New York: Rowman & Littlefield.

Yancey, George and Judith Butler. 2015. "What's Wrong With 'All Lives Matter'?" Editorial. *Opinonator* (blog), *New York Times*. January 12, 2015. https://opinionator.blogs.nytimes.com.

Yoon, In-Jin. 2007. *On My Own: Korean Businesses and Race Relations in America*. Chicago: University of Chicago Press.

Young, Iris Marion. 1980. "Throwing Like a Girl: A Phenomenology of Feminine Body Comportment, Motility, and Spatiality." In *On Female Body Experience: "Throwing Like a Girl" and Other Essays*, 137–156. Oxford: Oxford University Press.

Young, James O. and Conrad G. Brunk. 2009. *The Ethics of Cultural Appropriation*. Malden, NY: Blackwell Publishing.

Zdatny, Steven. 2006. *Fashion, Work, and Politics in Modern France*. New York: Palgrave Macmillan.

Zinn, Maxine Baca, Lynn Weber Cannon, Elizabeth Higginbotham, and Bonnie Thornton Dill. 1986. "The Costs of Exclusionary Practices in Women's Studies." *Signs: Journal of Women in Culture and Society* 11 (2): 290–303.

Zola, Irving. 1972. "Medicine as an Institution of Social Control." *The Sociological Review* 20 (4): 487–504.

INDEX

Page numbers in *italics* indicate Figures

ABOUT THE AUTHOR

CHELSEA MARY ELISE JOHNSON (she/her) is a sociologist and applied researcher specializing in designing trusted, safe, and equitable online user experiences. Her journey into research began at Spelman College, where she was introduced to feminism through writers like Audre Lorde and Patricia Hill Collins. She went on to study the politics of race, class, gender, and beauty at the University of Southern California, where she earned her PhD in sociology and gender studies in 2019. Her writing on race, gender, and embodiment has appeared in *Cultural History of Hair, Sociology of Sport Journal, Liber, Women's Review of Books, Ms. Magazine, CRWN, The Conversation,* and more. When not researching or writing, you'll find Chelsea on long walks with her daughter, Sloane.